■ SUPERSENSE ■

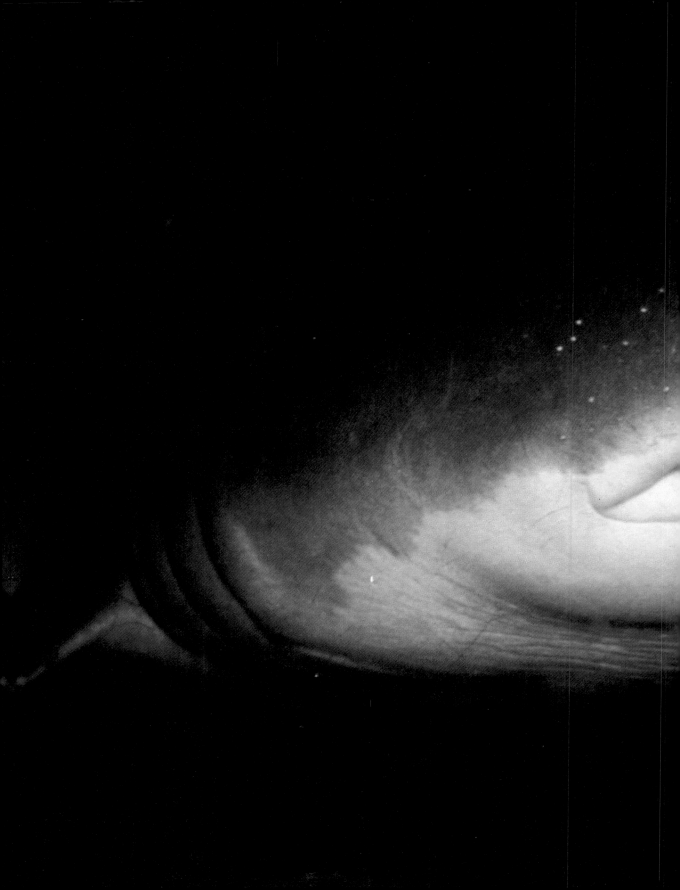

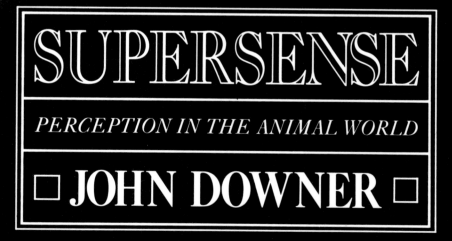

SUPERSENSE

PERCEPTION IN THE ANIMAL WORLD

☐ JOHN DOWNER ☐

BBC BOOKS

TO SARA

ACKNOWLEDGEMENTS

This book is a companion to the BBC Television series *Supersense*. Both projects
have only been possible because of the pioneering research of many scientists
throughout the world. Over the last two years many of them have generously
given guidance and information about their work. I am indebted to them all.
In particular I would like to thank Robin Baker, Roger Coles, Adrijanus
Kalmijn, Margaret Klinowska, Arthur Myrberg, Julian Partridge, Joyce Poole,
Graham Martin and Douglas Quine for their influential advice. Mike Land, John
Lythgoe, Gillian Sales and Max Westby deserve special thanks for also reading
extracts from the book and weeding out misconceptions.
I am also grateful for the constant support from the *Supersense* team. Mark
Jacobs and Nigel Marven, the two assistant producers, contributed countless
ideas and encouragement. Andrew Kitchener and Rupert Barrington helped
with the series research and Liz Appleby, my assistant, gave me considerable
support and valiantly deciphered my scrawl.

Previous page: Sand tiger shark

Pages 6–7: Alpine choughs

Published by BBC Books,
a division of BBC Enterprises Limited,
Woodlands, 80 Wood Lane, London W12 OTT
First published 1988
© John Downer 1988
ISBN 0 563 20660 8
Set in 11 on 13½ point Bembo
Printed and bound in Great Britain by Butler & Tanner Ltd,
Frome and London

■ CONTENTS

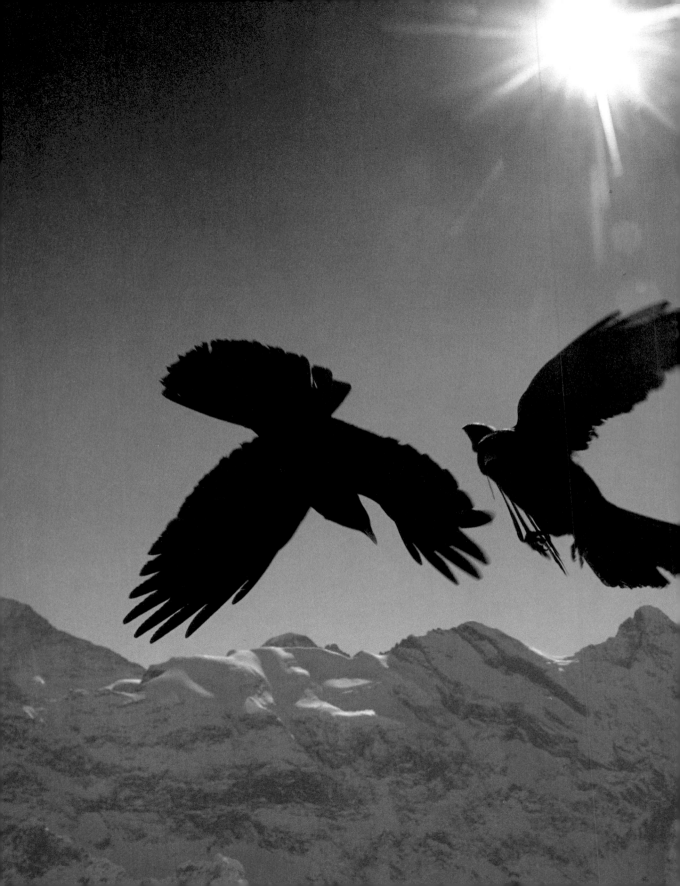

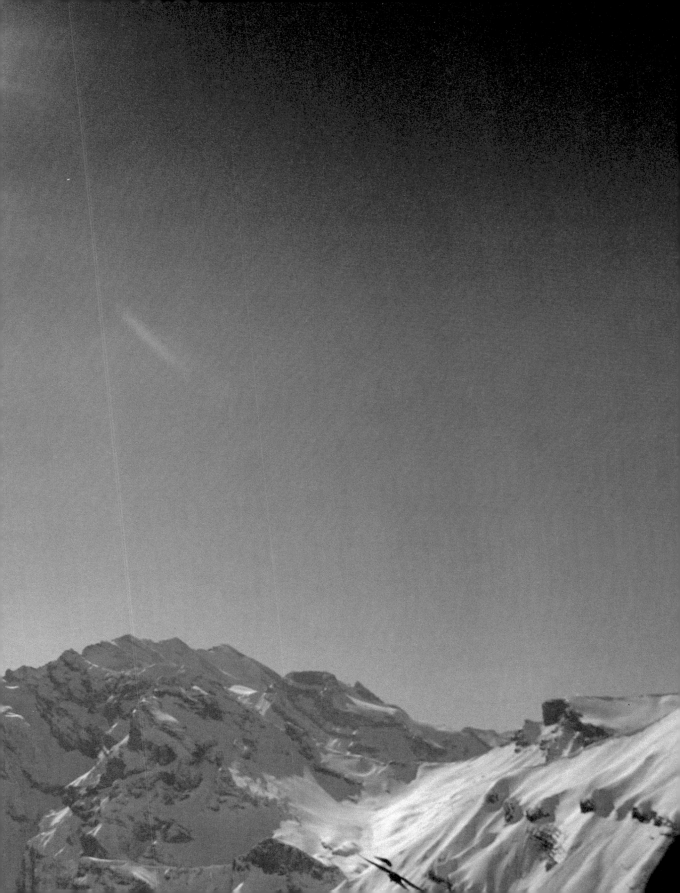

INTRODUCTION

For centuries, man has thought of himself as the most highly evolved form of life on earth, using his five senses to build up a composite and highly complex picture of the world around him. Confident in our own superiority over the rest of the animal kingdom, it has rarely occurred to us to question how other creatures perceive the world. But are we really so superior? One of the aims the BBC television series, *Supersense*, and this book which accompanies it, was to challenge that assumption.

We pride ourselves, for example, on having acute eyesight, yet the eyesight of birds of prey, swooping down on their victims with uncanny precision, far exceeds ours. This was vividly brought home to us during the filming of *Supersense*. Our plan was to simulate the view of a vulture by mounting a camera on a model aircraft: we would wait near a fresh lion kill until the vultures started soaring, and then fly the model aircraft among them as they descended on the carcass. Each morning we scanned the sky, hoping to spy the vultures gathering above us. However, by the time we had spotted the first speck through our high-powered binoculars, the vulture was already descending. Within seconds, the formerly empty sky was full with birds plummeting onto the carcass. Although we could barely make out the carcass 300 metres away from us, the vultures, high above the reach of our binocular-aided vision, could see it clearly.

We tend to think of animal vision only in terms of that part of the spectrum of light which *we* can see; and yet we know that the spectrum extends far beyond this. Incredibly there are animals, such as the pit viper, that can see the infra-red part of the spectrum. Many insects can detect ultraviolet light, while the vision of the common goldfish ranges from ultraviolet to far-red: achievements that we have only been able to equal in recent years with the development of sophisticated electronic equipment.

Sound, too, possibly the second most important sense to man, covers a range far greater than that which we can hear. As we filmed the elephants in Amboseli National Park, East Africa, the animals sometimes wandered so close to us that we could hear their trunks ripping the grass and their stomachs churning. These animals were also communicating with each other, but we were only able to catch the deep rumbles which are the upper harmonies of their conversation. Most of their communications were lost to us, being below our hearing range.

Above our hearing, bats flit around in total darkness, judging their distance from objects by emitting high-pitched bursts of sound and timing how long it takes for the echo of the sound to bounce back. Again, it has taken years of painstaking research to enable us to emulate devices which other creatures make regular use of in their everyday lives.

We are all familiar with the way in which our sense of smell (and therefore taste, for the two are closely linked) is impaired when we have a heavy cold. Smell is also an important factor in identification: in common with many other animals, we recognise things – and even other members of our own species – by their unique personal smell. But many animals take this even further: creatures as different from each other as salmon and pigeons may even navigate by smell, detecting minute changes in the concentration of certain chemicals in the water or odours wafting through the air.

In producing *Supersense*, the animal that I personally have become closest to is a European green-winged teal, which follows me everywhere. As I write, this duck is setting at my feet. Even so, I am continually aware that the teal is experiencing the world through senses very different from my own. It is impossible to creep up on the duck, because its 360 degree vision takes in the slightest movement anywhere around it. It combines this wrap-around view with the ability to pick out any detail which might be significant in a duck's life. When leaving the house one day, the bird suddenly cocked its head and looked up at the sky. By peering hard in the same direction, I could just make out the faint flicker of a distant plane. The duck had instantly spied this tiny speck which might signify a flying predator.

These examples of animal senses are relatively easy for us to comprehend as they are not too far removed from our own experience. But the animal world contains many things which may strike us as being strange or even inexplicable. How do birds know when to migrate and, even more puzzling, how do they find their way? Why do some animals – and even plants – have a reputation for being able to predict bad weather? What causes the periodic swarming – at 13 or 17-year intervals – of cicadas?

Luckily, many scientists have started to make the leaps of imagination required to answer these questions. Through their researches, I know that many of these events are the result of creatures picking up subtle cues from the environment which we, with all our 'hi-tech' equipment, are quite unable to detect. Our mistake in the past has been to assume that because other forms of life perceive things differently from us, they are necessarily inferior: they are not. Pioneering scientific work is now opening up the immense diversity of sensory worlds experienced by other creatures: extraordinary worlds which we may never be able to enter, but which we can at least start to appreciate through our awareness of animal 'supersenses'.

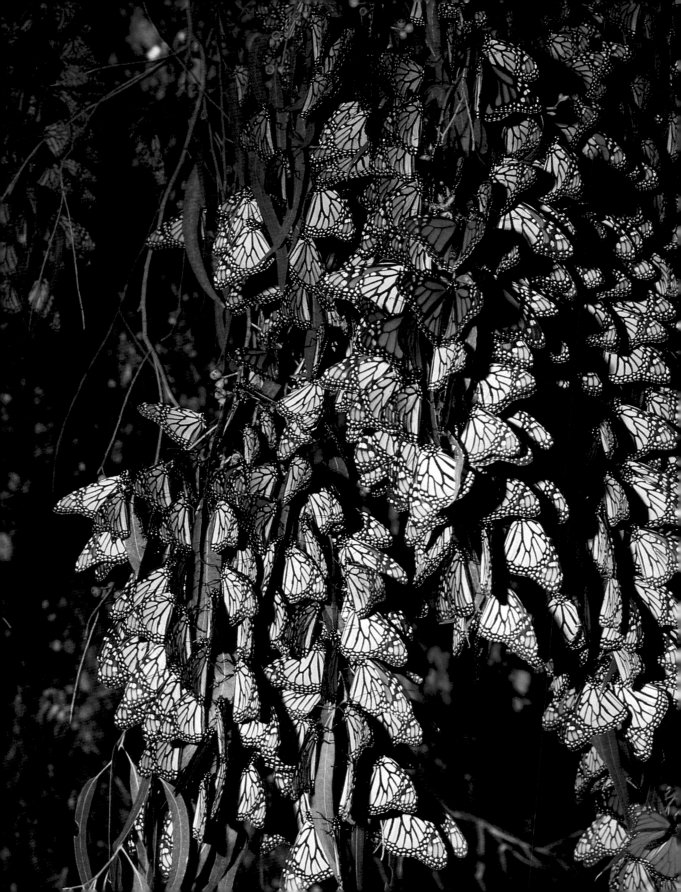

SIXTH SENSE

We experience our surroundings through the five main senses of sight, hearing, touch, taste and smell. For many centuries people assumed that other animals had a similar, if perhaps more limited, view of the world. Any strange or inexplicable behaviour, both in humans and in the natural world, was put down to some supernatural sixth sense. Animals showing special powers were regarded as magical; some were even worshipped.

One of the longest mythological pedigrees belongs to the snake, which has been the subject of both loathing and reverence. Its reputation was partly due to its grotesque appearance, and also to the snake's uncanny ability to appear out of nowhere and deliver a lethal strike, sometimes in total darkness. The shark's prodigious hunting skills earned it a similar position among oceanic peoples. Other animals were credited with more benign talents, such as being able to forecast the weather or to predict earthquakes.

Research is showing that many animals actually do possess a sixth sense but this is a natural 'supersense', rather than anything supernatural. Another example is the numbfish which Pliny the Elder wrote about in the first century AD. He described with horror this fish's ability to paralyse anyone who came near it. Electricity – the key to this mystery – was not discovered until seventeen centuries later. Science has now revealed that some fish use electricity to stun, to find prey and even to 'see' around them.

Such animals may appear magical to us because we tend to cling to our own heavily filtered reality. Before journeying into the sensory worlds of other animals we need to discard this restricted view. We react to cues which are significant to us, such as light, sounds and smells, while ignoring a wide variety of other stimuli. Like us, each creature responds selectively to cues from its environment, only tuning into those which are important to it. Some have the same senses as us but may utilise them very differently. Others perceive the world in ways difficult for us to even imagine.

HEAT SENSORS

We can judge the temperature of the air around us, and any object we touch, through nerve endings in the skin. There are spots sensitive to either heat or cold between 1 and 5 millimetres apart all over the skin. This system is fairly crude, though, and we are bad at discerning small differences in temperature. We can even be misled, for if a cold spot is touched with a warm needle it can produce a sensation of coldness.

In contrast, the turkey-like incubator bird, or mallee fowl, of Australia has a very accurate natural thermometer in its bill. This bird is so named because it incubates its eggs in a mound of rotting vegetation. Every few minutes the cock tests the temperature of the mound: if it falls below 33 degrees Celsius he adds more compost, while if it rises above 33 degrees he makes a vent in the mound to cool the eggs. In this way, the eggs are maintained at the optimum temperature.

Being warm-blooded animals, both incubator birds and ourselves automatically adjust our own body temperatures to keep our bodily processes working smoothly. A number of animals are able to take advantage of this body heat. Bugs are very sensitive to the slight change in temperature caused by the approach of a potential host. Bugs use their antennae to detect blood heat, while a tick will sink its proboscis into any liquid at blood heat, even water.

Until recently, it was thought that a mammal would be unable to use this method to find food because its own body heat would blot out the host's. However, that favourite creature of horror movies – the vampire bat – has solved this problem. Its face has a strange convoluted patch of skin known as a nose-leaf, which contains heat-sensitive areas. The nose-leaf is separated from the bat's body warmth by a layer of tissue, causing it to be 9 degrees Celsius colder. Isolated in this way, the heat-sensitive areas can detect the warmth of an animal from about 16 centimetres away. In concert with other senses, the bat's nose-leaf allows it to find prey and helps it to discriminate between, say, a cold hoof and the warmer blood-filled tissue further up the leg.

Remarkable though the vampire bat's skill is, it pales into insignificance besides that of another legendary animal, the snake. When a bat detects heat it is actually sensing the infra-red radiation given off by a warm body. We experience this radiation when we enjoy the heat of a glowing fire or the sun. In common with most other animals, including ourselves, the eyes of most snakes can only respond to the radiation which we call light. However, two families of snake have also developed such sophisticated infra-red detectors that they can effectively 'see' their prey in total darkness.

Some boids, including the boa constrictor, python and anaconda, have a row of up to thirteen heat-sensitive organs. The pit vipers, such as the rattlesnake and the mocassin, have a heat-sensitive organ on either side of the face between the eyes and the nostrils. In a full-grown pit viper, each organ is about 0.5 centimetres deep, and always faces forward. The opening to the organ is only a few millimetres in diameter, and so it acts rather like a pin-hole camera, but one that focuses infra-red heat radiation instead of light.

The infra-red radiation is projected onto a membrane stretched across the organ. The membrane contains a grid of 7000 nerve endings which respond to tiny variations in temperature to produce a heat picture. The system is so sensitive that the organs can detect changes in temperature as small as 0.003 degrees Celsius, while they can respond to such changes in an incredible 35 milliseconds – many hundreds of times faster than any human-made device.

The information from the membrane is passed to the area of the brain that deals with vision, and it is analysed in a similar way to signals from the eyes. The resolution of the infra-red detectors is much poorer than that of the eyes, and so the heat image is rather crude. However, it is detailed enough to reveal any warm-blooded creatures in the vicinity. During the day, a well-camouflaged animal may escape the eyes of a snake, but it will be given away by the halo of its infra-red radiation. Even when all light fades, the ghostly image of the prey's body heat continues.

Both pythons and pit vipers also have heat sensors in the mouth. As the snake closes in for the kill, its mouth sensors guide it with deadly accuracy.

At such times, possessing body heat is fatal, but being warm-blooded also has many advantages. In particular, it allows animals to continue their activities whatever the weather. Generally, though, all animals try to avoid bad weather, and, in the past, their habits were used as a natural weather gauge.

WEATHER FORECASTING

Weather prediction is vital to the success of farming and other activities, and for centuries people have watched the natural world closely and used it as a guide. Over the years, a vast folklore has built up, much of it linking the behaviour of plants and animals to the weather. Cows lying down heralding rain and swallows flying high signalling good weather are two of the many indications that people have followed.

As the science of meteorology has advanced towards the computerised forecasts we receive today, this folklore has been treated with increasing suspicion, or forgotten. In parts of Provence, though, farmers still keep green tree frogs under glass bells so that their croaking can warn of rain, and many people keep a piece of dried seaweed, claiming that it is as accurate as the human meteorologist's forecasts. In fact, the texture of the seaweed does vary according to the humidity of the air. Traditionally, other plants have also been regarded as natural barometers. Many, such as marigolds, corn sow thistles and sunflowers, only open their flowers in fine weather. Their flowerheads even follow the course of the sun like satellite tracking dishes. Before rain, these and many other flowers close up to protect their pollen-bearing anthers. The scarlet pimpernel is so sensitive that it is often known as the Poor Man's Weather Glass. Chickweed and convolvulus are similar flower barometers. Other plants, such as clovers and wood sorrel, react to the approach of bad weather by folding their leaves.

These weather-sensitive plants respond to changes in temperature, humidity and

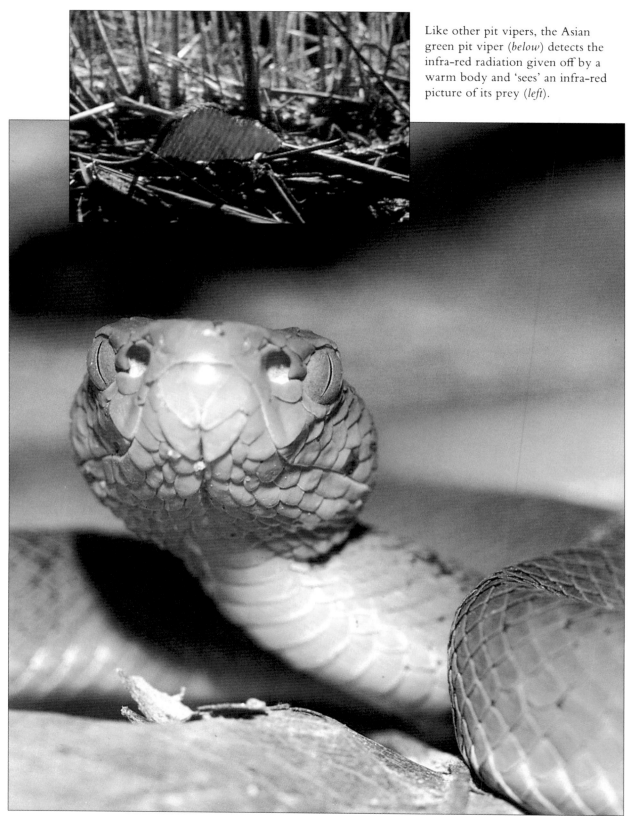

Like other pit vipers, the Asian green pit viper (*below*) detects the infra-red radiation given off by a warm body and 'sees' an infra-red picture of its prey (*left*).

light. Research is showing that many animals respond to other weather cues.

In a rainstorm enormous electrical discharges occur in clouds and become visible in the lightning bolts that discharge to the ground. These electrical disturbances create electromagnetic waves which spread through the atmosphere for hundreds of kilometres. Any animal that could detect these waves would have a reliable indicator of weather changes ahead.

Bees have a reputation for foretelling the weather. Before a thunderstorm, they become increasingly agitated and return to the hive in large numbers. When subjected to artificial electric fields they show similar behaviour. At high intensities they will even remove broods from cells or sting each other to death. Hamsters also show a strong reaction to artificial electric fields, and will change the position of their nests to avoid its effects.

Such animals are likely to be equally sensitive to the electromagnetic waves created by a storm. They may also be sensitive to static electrical charges in the air. Before a storm the air becomes charged with positive ions. In mammals this is known to influence the concentration of a brain hormone known as serotonin, which in turn controls sleep and other metabolic processes. This could account for the weather sensitivity of some people who show either depression before a storm, or pains in joints and injuries.

Much more dramatic are the large-scale movements of birds. If migrating birds are caught up in a storm, or blown off course, it can be disastrous for, even undisturbed, these vast journeys stretch them to the limit. Birds occasionally encounter bad weather, but usually they are successful at predicting favourable conditions. When migrating to the northern hemisphere they choose a time when the atmospheric pressure is falling, the temperature is rising and the winds are blowing northwards. They leave the northern hemisphere's autumn when the pressure is rising, the temperature falling and the winds are blowing southwards.

It is thought that they are able to do this partly by measuring pressure, just as we rely on atmospheric pressure readings from barometers to forecast the weather. Tests have shown that pigeons and ducks have accurate in-built barometers, capable of detecting minute air pressure changes. Indeed, pigeons are so sensitive that they can detect the difference in pressure between one floor of a building and another. The birds' pressure sense could be used not only to predict the weather, but also to maintain the correct altitude when in flight.

Certain ants, such as the common black ant found in the garden, use weather cues for a very different purpose – to ensure successful mating. These ants produce winged sexual forms in late summer. The wingless workers tend these flying males and queens in the nest, sometimes for several weeks. Meanwhile the workers continually monitor the temperature and humidity, waiting for the conditions that signal perfect mating weather. When a period of stable, anticyclonic weather arrives, the workers release a chemical into the air which stimulates the males and queens to emerge simultaneously from nests over many square kilometres. The males and queens rise up in a nuptial flight and mate on the wing. A fraction of this huge number of ants satiates the predators, and the majority of queens survive to found new colonies.

THE TREMBLING EARTH

If someone drops a pebble a metre away from a ghost crab, the crab will instantly run to the spot. It locates its food by vibrations and is attracted to anything which generates the right sort of disturbance.

Cat flea pupae use vibrations in a slightly different way. They lie dormant, usually in carpets, until they feel the faint tremble that indicates a person or a cat passing, and then rapidly emerge. They leap on to their host, guided in the final stages by the host's body heat and the carbon dioxide in its breath. The pupae can remain dormant for months, or even years, waiting for the right vibrations, which is why a person moving into a previously empty house may suffer a plague of fleas.

Another household pest, the cockroach, is even more sensitive. When the vibration detector in its leg was tested in a laboratory, it could perceive movements as small as 2000 times the diameter of a hydrogen atom. Leaf-cutter ants seem to be able to detect equally tiny vibrations. If one of their underground galleries collapses, the buried ants tap out a call for help. Other leaf-cutter ants can detect this signal through 5 centimetres of earth, and rush to rescue the trapped workers.

Ground-borne vibrations are particularly useful for communicating through the earth and many subterranean species make use of them. When termites leave the nest to forage on dead plant material, they can remain hidden by building tunnels from the nest to the food supplies. However, they are still vulnerable to predators that dig. At the slightest sign of disturbance, the termites drum out a warning on the earth, which causes the whole foraging party to disappear up the tunnels back to the nest.

Small burrowing rodents, known as mole-rats, live in the drier parts of Africa. They use their chisel-like teeth to dig out a complex system of burrows, and solidify the ceilings by pressing the soil with their flattened heads. Some live communally, while others live alone for much of the year. The solitary species use the head to thump out messages, and each species has its own rhythmic code, which may help individuals identify each other in underground encounters. The thumps are also used to maintain a territory and attract a mate. Even above ground, vibrations can be used for communication. Female brown plant hoppers send a signal to their mates by beating their abdomen against a leaf twenty times each second. The males respond with a drumming four times as fast. By alternating these messages, the males and females soon find each other.

Vibrations do not pass only through the ground. In fact, they travel far better in water, and animals of ponds, lakes, rivers and seas have evolved ingenious ways of utilising them.

RIPPLE DETECTORS

Frenzied swarms of small black beetles can often be seen on the surface of still ponds and lakes. These aptly named whirligig beetles spin round continually, creating a dizzy display which confuses potential predators, and yet the beetles appear never to collide. Each manages to avoid the others by means of a special divided antenna, one part of which rests on the water surface. The slightest vibration of the surface is detected by the antenna, and the whirligig can distinguish between its own ripples and the myriad ripples produced by other whirligigs.

The beetle's ripples bounce off any object breaking the surface of the water, and the whirligig can avoid such obstacles by sensing the reflected ripples. Another clue is provided by the fact that the water surface curves when it meets an object. The whirligig sometimes moves so fast that it overtakes its own ripples, and then any slight slope in the surface alerts it to an obstacle. The beetle's antenna also helps it to locate prey by sensing the tell-tale vibrations of any small insect which falls onto the surface.

The water strider finds its food in a similar way, and grabs its prey between its short front legs. The insect also communicates through ripples, using its legs to tap on the surface of the water. Its message proclaims its sex, for male striders generate a barrage of ninety ripples a minute, while females tap only ten times a minute. Below the surface, other animals are also tuning into water movements.

UNDERWATER VIBRATIONS

Another common pond insect, the water boatman or backswimmer, lies just below the surface of the water and senses the ripples created by prey through special organs in the first segments of the legs. These organs respond to minute movements of the claws pressed against the water surface. Detecting water movements helps many insects of fast-flowing streams to maintain their position, and it alerts aquatic leeches to the approach of animals which might provide a meal of blood. However, sensitivity to water movements is most developed in underwater vertebrates.

A remarkable fish, *Astyanax fasciatus*, lives in the cold inky blackness of a Mexican cave. With no use for its eyes, it has lost its sight and yet it manages to locate shelter, a mate, and even food. To find its way around, the fish relies on a system found in many other fish and some amphibians.

These animals have what are called lateral line organs along their head and body. Each organ consists of sensitive hairs attached to a jelly-like rod, which bends in the

For centuries people have reported observing strange animal behaviour before earthquakes and volcanic eruptions. Cats leave villages taking their kittens with them, horses stampede, birds sing at the wrong time of day, cows break out of barns and rats appear in the street in broad daylight. It seems that the animals may be able to detect electrical changes in the air, as rocks are stressed.

Some animals may also hear the low rumbles of a quake long before they become audible to humans. Birds and elephants are both sensitive to such low-frequency sound and will react before an earthquake hits. Many animals such as snakes are also acutely sensitive to vibration and may well feel the tiny pre-tremors that often precede a quake.

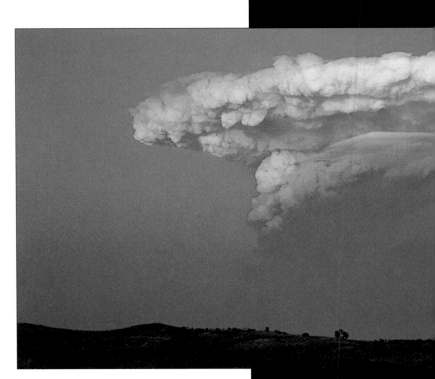

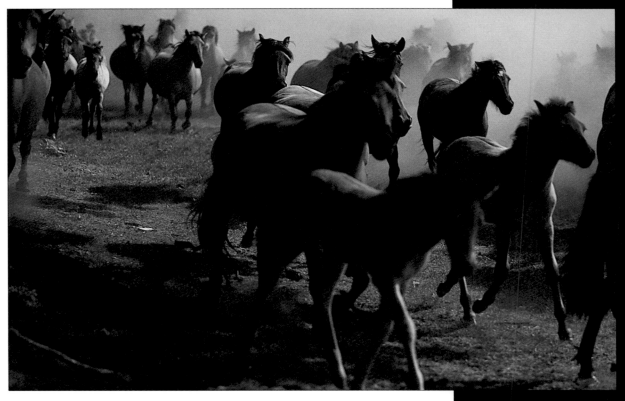

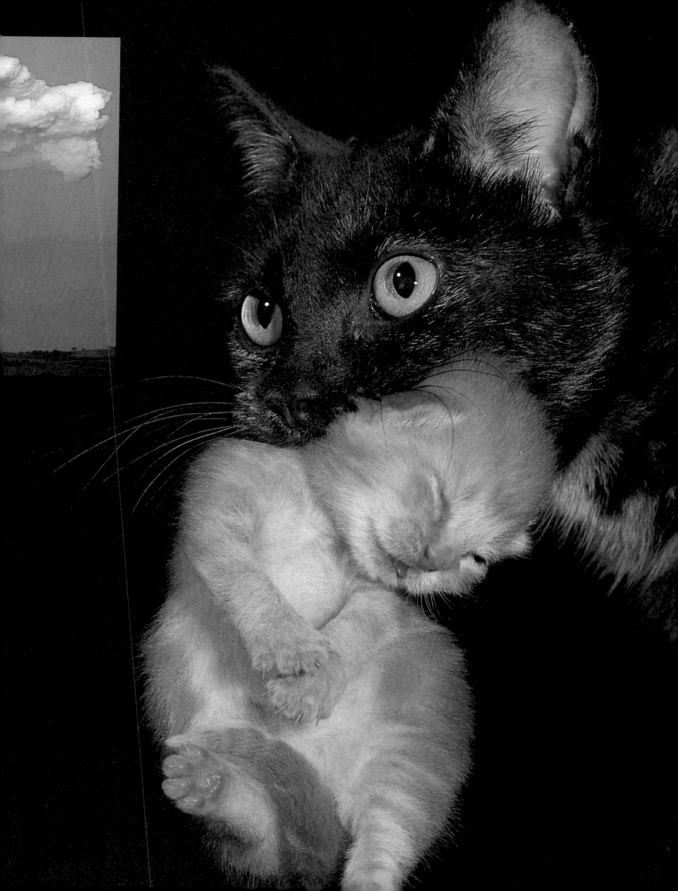

direction of any water movement. Disturbances caused by predators, prey or other creatures are sensed by these organs. Because they are arranged along the animal, each of the organs receives a slightly different impression of a disturbance, allowing the animal to locate its source and build up a picture of its surroundings.

The detail of the picture can be masked, however, by water currents or the movements of the animal itself. Many fish have found a neat solution to this problem. Their lateral line organs are buried in canals which run along the head and body, and open into the water through pores. Using this refined system, a fish can actually improve detail by swimming fast. The disturbances it creates bounce off objects, which are then sensed by the water waves they reflect.

As well as building up a picture of the surroundings, the lateral line allows shoaling fish, such as herrings, to maintain their position in the group. This system is also used by fish to find food, and it is often tuned to the body vibrations of prey. One Antarctic fish, *Pagothenia*, is irresistibly drawn to shrimps, which vibrate at 40 hertz (cycles per second). In fact, the fish will come to anything generating this frequency, even an artificially vibrating sphere.

The ease with which predatory fish can be misled has sinister implications for humans. Hunting sharks are particularly sensitive to vibrations of 200 hertz, and this is the frequency produced by the rotary blades of a hovering helicopter. So an air-sea rescue mission may accidentally sound a dinner bell for nearby sharks.

AIR-CURRENT DETECTORS

When a strong to moderate wind blows against our skin we can usually feel the wind's direction, although we often rely more on the direction in which trees or smoke are being blown. Even in a light wind, we can sometimes gauge direction by wetting a finger and sensing which side of the finger cools most quickly through evaporation of the water by the wind. However, a scorpion can detect air moving at 0.072 kilometres per hour – 100 times slower than a light breeze on the Beaufort scale.

The scorpion's natural anemometers are special hairs on its pincers. Spiders have similar hairs on their legs. Each hair vibrates mainly in one direction and responds most to air moving in that direction. By sensing the movements of different hairs, the animal can tell the direction of any air currents. As it moves, the scorpion relies on information from air passing over its hairs to keep it on a straight course.

For flying insects, accurate knowledge of air movements is vital for flight control. The bee gauges its speed of flight from the amount its antennae are bent outwards by the air rushing past. If they bend too much, the bee responds by moving its wings less strongly and so maintains an optimum speed.

For insects such as locusts, which migrate over vast distances, it is even more important to fly at an economical speed. In addition to using its antennae, the locust has a patch of hairs on its head, which are sensitive to air currents. As the locust flies, the passage of air causes the antennae to bend outwards and the locust reduces speed by beating its wings less strongly. The passing air currents have the opposite effect on the hairs, stimulating the insect to fly faster. These two systems working in opposition seem to give the locust very fine speed control.

If insects judged their speed solely on the basis of the speed of the air moving past, they would remain stationary when attempting to fly into the wind. In fact, the insect's eyes assess its speed relative to the ground, and this visual information has overall control. If the ground is moving slowly, the insect moves its antennae inwards and so beats its wings more strongly, while if the ground is moving by too fast, it compensates by moving the antennae outwards. In this way, the insect can make progress even against a light headwind.

All flying animals need such control, including those masters of the air, the birds. Migrating birds display great sensitivity to the direction and force of air currents, changing altitude frequently to find the best conditions, and yet for many years their sensors have eluded detection. Recent research indicates that the secret may lie in their feathers.

Birds have two main types of feather, contour and down, plus tiny hair-like feathers called filoplumes which lie alongside each contour feather. The filoplumes move with the contour feathers, and have small touch receptors at their bases. These hairs therefore feed the bird continuous information about the position of each contour feather. This system helps the bird keep its plumage in shape, and any ruffled feathers are quickly preened back into place. It seems that the filoplumes may also be used to sense the air currents around the bird's body. For example, blowing on the breast feathers of a bird of prey causes it to stretch its wings out.

This theory was tested out on small finches called siskins. Like many small birds on a long-distance flight, siskins save energy by interspersing their flapping flight with short periods of gliding. When siskins had their breast feathers temporarily covered, the speed of their flight increased and they did not glide at all. This indicates the importance of free movement of the feathers in flight control.

An even more vital skill in long migratory flights is accurate navigation, and birds have another special sense to aid them in this.

MAGNETIC ANIMALS

In 1975, some strange bacteria were discovered in sediment at Woodhole, Massachusetts. Unlike any organisms seen before, they moved in a direction determined by the Earth's

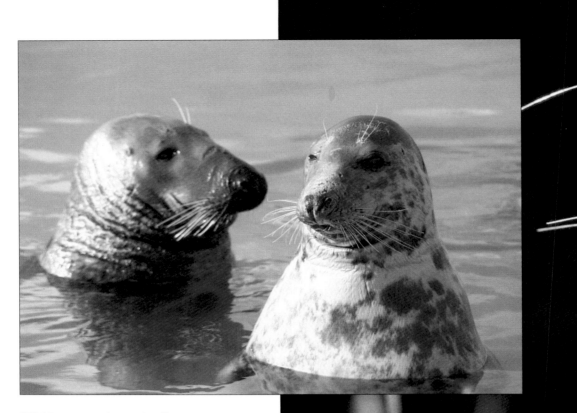

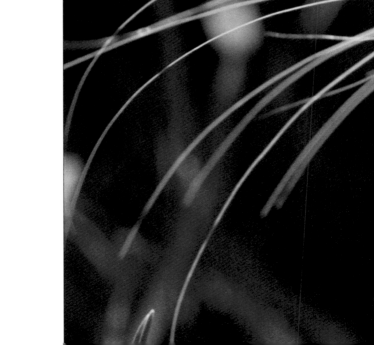

Whiskers extend an animal's sense of touch beyond the body. The whiskers are formed from stiff modified hairs. When these are bent, the follicle at the base of each hair detects both the direction and speed of the bending.

A cat without whiskers is very unsure in the dark and has difficulty in negotiating narrow corridors. The information from the whiskers travels along the same path as information from the eyes, and the cat's brain seems to use the two systems together to build up a three-dimensional view of its surroundings.

Seals, such as this grey seal, rely on whiskers to locate fish. As blind seals are often found to be well-fed, it seems that this sense is more important than vision. The whiskers are thought to respond to nearby water movement.

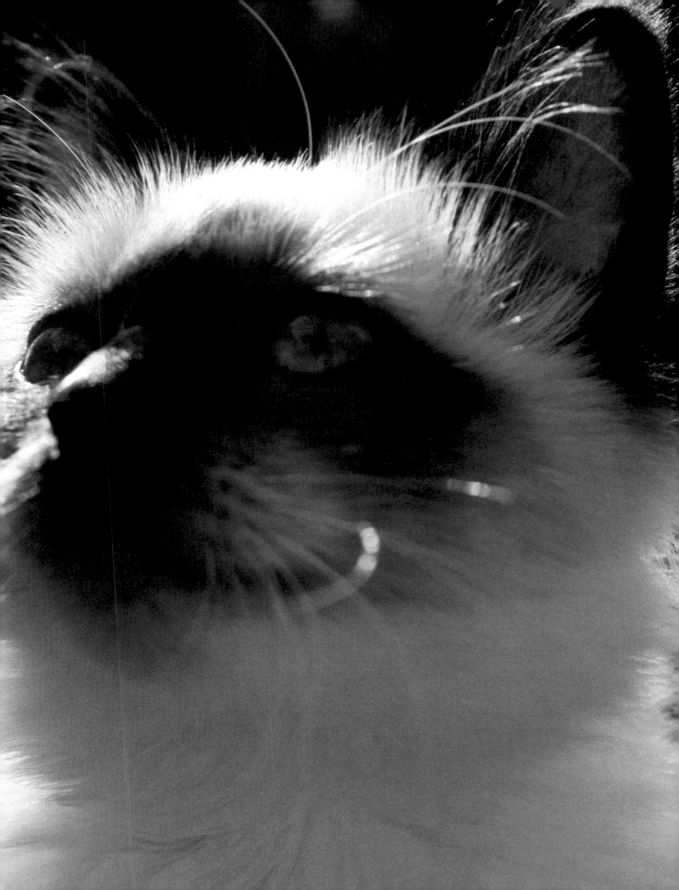

magnetic field. Further investigation revealed that each bacterium contained a chain of crystals of an iron compound, known as lodestone or magnetite, which always points towards the Earth's magnetic poles. For centuries, bars of magnetite were used by sailors to guide them across the unvarying expanse of the oceans, and it is only fairly recently that manufactured substances have replaced this naturally occurring ore in compasses.

At Woodhole, the Earth's magnetism pulls downwards and during the bacteria's short life of an hour or so, they move in the direction of this force. It is thought that, because bacteria are so tiny, the Earth's gravity has little effect on them and they need their miniature magnets to guide them into the sediment.

Since this discovery, magnetite has been found in many other animals, including the familiar honeybee. The magnetite particles on the honeybee's abdomen may be responsible for the bee's sensitivity to the Earth's magnetic field. Experiments show that bees can be trained to come to sugar solutions in response to an artificial magnetic field. Their magnetic sense also seems to influence the bees' comb building. A beehive contains a number of parallel vertical combs. When a swarm of bees leave to found a new colony, they tend to build combs with the same orientation, say east–west, as the combs in their parent hive. The orientation of the combs can be changed, however, by applying an artificial magnetic field, showing that magnetism is an important cue.

Magnetism may also be used during one of the longest migrations in the insect world. Each autumn, the monarch butterflies in North America undertake a vast journey of up to 4000 kilometres southwards. Those on the western side of the continent travel down to California, while the eastern population of roughly 100 million butterflies overwinters in a small area of central Mexico. The butterflies which fly south are several generations removed from those which flew north in the previous spring. Their knowledge of the migration route is, therefore, inherited. Like many butterflies, they appear to use the position of the sun as a guide to compass direction. However, they are unlikely to be able to navigate sufficiently accurately using this cue alone. Of all the butterflies tested so far, monarchs contain the greatest amount of magnetite, and they probably also use the Earth's magnetic field to accomplish their feat.

Magnetite occurs in many other creatures incuding turtles, tuna, mice and birds. At one time, the discovery of magnetite in an animal's tissue was thought to indicate that the animal had a magnetic sense. However, this substance has been found in so many different tissues of such a wide variety of animals, that there is now some doubt about its role and the quest for a natural magnetic detector is continuing. Whatever the mechanism employed, many creatures certainly can detect the Earth's magnetic field, and a magnetic sense may even explain some of the mysteries of bird migration.

At one time, people thought that birds transformed themselves into other creatures during the winter. The discovery of the true facts only increased people's fascination, for birds' arduous migrations demand phenomenal navigation skills. Many experiments were performed to try to solve this puzzle.

Some research indicated that, like early sailors, birds find their way using the sun and the stars. However, a bird with impaired vision can complete its journey successfully. Other investigations suggested that smells or even sounds may be used as guides, but, again, birds lacking one of these senses can still cope. In fact, just as we rely on many senses to guide us, birds probably use a wide range of cues in navigation. Underlying all of these seems to be a highly developed magnetic sense.

It has been suggested that young birds use their magnetic sense to orient a compass based on the sun and the stars. As they mature, they rely on this celestial compass, falling back on the Earth's magnetism when visibility is poor.

Similarly, we use artificial compasses to follow a course. Most of us assume that without these we could not detect the Earth's magnetic field. However, tests have been carried out at Manchester University, England, to find out whether we also possess a natural magnetic sense. In one of the experiments, a group of students were blindfolded and then taken on a coachride. Half of the students had strong magnets on their heads, while the rest wore non-magnetic metal bars. When the coach stopped and the students were asked to point to home, those without magnets performed significantly better than those with magnets. This suggested that the artificial magnets were interfering with a natural magnetic sense. Other experiments led to similar conclusions but, unfortunately, tests performed elsewhere have failed to confirm these findings. So, although it seems likely that we too have a magnetic sense, this is as yet unproven.

With very sensitive equipment, tiny variations in the Earth's magnetic field can be detected all over the surface. This information has been used to draw up magnetic maps, similar in style to contour maps. Some animals appear to have a highly developed magnetic sense and use magnetic variations to find their way around.

MAGNETIC TRAILS

Large groups of whales occasionally swim ashore and lie stranded on the beach, unable to move their huge bulks back into the sea. Accounts of such mass strandings date back centuries. Yet until recently there was no explanation for this bizarre behaviour, other than that it was probably due to a breakdown of some unknown navigation system. Then, records of strandings in Britain and the United States were plotted against magnetic maps. These magnetic maps plot the variations in intensity of the Earth's magnetic field caused by differences in the underlying rocks. The variations are represented by contour lines so that areas of high magnetism appear as hills and areas of low magnetism show up as valleys. Most strandings were found to occur where the 'valleys' ran directly from the sea to the shore.

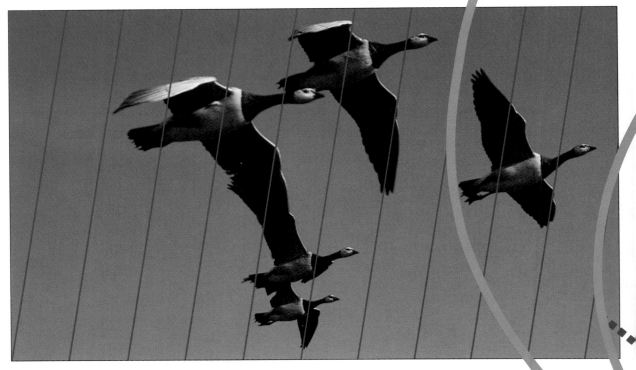

■ Migrating birds use a magnetic sense to find their way, backing up information they receive from the sun and stars. They rely on the fact that the Earth is a giant magnet and that magnetic lines of force spread out around it just as they do around a bar magnet. A migrant finds compass direction by sensing the angle these invisible lines of force make with its body as it flies through them. This is known as the angle of dip. For northern migrants, such as barnacle geese, the lines of force are angled towards the bird as they fly south and away from them as they fly north. At the Equator the lines of force are horizontal and, in relation to the bird's body, they are angled neither to the north or south. Birds such as flamingoes, which fly over this region on their migration route, have difficulty using magnetic information to find their compass direction, and have to rely on other cues.

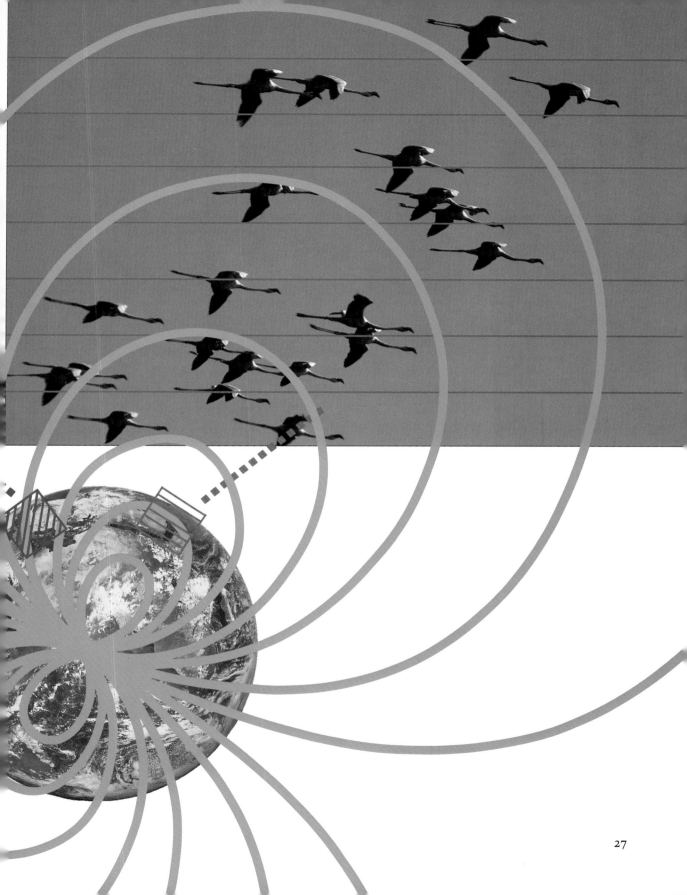

This sensational finding suggests that whales navigate by following a magnetic map of the ocean floor. On land, magnetic variations are very irregular, and anyway there are many physical features to act as a guide. There are no landmarks in the vast, dark ocean, but there are very regular magnetic variations. Magnetic hills and valleys stretch for huge distances across the ocean floor, and the whales appear to use the magnetic contour lines as invisible 'roads'. What method they use to detect such minute variations in magnetism remains a mystery, however.

Mass strandings usually involve whales which migrate over long distances. The more sedentary dolphins and porpoises seldom run into these difficulties. They presumbly become familiar with all the small local anomalies and so build up a much more detailed magnetic map of the area they live in.

Besides acting as an enormous magnet, the Earth's magnetic field has another useful property. It causes an electric current to flow through anything moving across it which can conduct electricity. This effect is used in the construction of dynamos. In a simple dynamo, an electric current is produced in a coil of wire by rotating the coil between opposite magnetic poles. When a fish swims across the Earth's magnetic field, like the coils of wire in a dynamo, tiny electric currents flow in its body. However, when the fish swims along the magnetic field, no current flows. If a fish was receptive enough to electricity to pick up any tiny currents induced in its body, they would provide an additional guide to the Earth's magnetic field. In fact, a number of underwater animals have sufficiently delicate electric sensors to detect induced currents and they appear to use them to orient themselves. Many certainly employ electricity to find prey. However, for this they lock into a different sort of electricity – that produced by the prey itself.

ELECTRIC SENSORS

We rely on electricity to keep our bodies working. The messages which travel through our nerves are carried by electrical impulses, and each muscle cell is activated by electricity. This body electricity is tapped to diagnose illnesses, for example, in electro-cardiographs of the heart and electroencephalograms of the brain.

Without such equipment, we cannot detect another person's electricity. Apart from our lack of sensitivity, the air is a very poor conductor of electricity. Currents do flow through water, however, and many underwater animals have developed the ability to tune into body electricity, particularly that of prey.

One such animal is the duckbill platypus. This is perhaps the strangest mammal of all, for not only does it lay eggs, but it also has a flattened bird-like bill. It lives in lakes and streams in Australia, hunting for shrimps often in murky water. This animal was shown to be sensitive to electricity by its behaviour towards batteries placed in its tank.

The platypus became very interested in a live 1.5v battery, investigating it with its bill, while it ignored a dead battery. This behaviour encouraged a more sophisticated experiment which involved placing two aluminium plates 3 metres apart in the tank. Tiny varying voltages were applied to the plates and the platypus's reactions showed that it could detect field strengths as low as a 500 millionth of a volt (0.05 microvolts) per centimetre. With this sensitivity it could easily detect a shrimp from over a metre away for these crustaceans generate tiny electrical fields of up to one thousandth of a volt (0.2–1 millivolt) per centimetre each time they flick their tails.

Further investigations revealed that the platypus's electric sensors lie within its bill, probably in glands which secrete a fluid to stop the sensors drying out on land. The odd flattened bill is also richly endowed with touch receptors, and the platypus seems to use its electric and touch senses together when searching for food.

So far, the ability to detect electricity has not been found in any other mammal. However, the talent has been discovered in the aquatic stages of some amphibians such as newts and caecilians. It is also widespread among fish.

Elasmobranchs, such as sharks and rays, are a very ancient group of fish that have a skeleton made of cartilage instead of bone. Like bony fish, they have lateral line organs which pick up the water movements made by prey. Their prey cannot escape detection by remaining still, however. These fish will detect the electricity made by the prey's muscles as it breathes, even if the prey hides in sediment on the ocean floor.

Their electric sensors, known as ampullae of Lorenzini, are arranged around the head. These jelly-filled tubes have electroreceptor cells at their ends, delicate enough to pick up the tiny discharges of the prey's body. The strongest electric sources are the muscle cells, and so the sharks and rays may perceive other fish as crude, shimmering images of hearts, gills and other muscles. They would be able to do so only from about a metre away, however, because even the muscles' discharges are tiny. So this electric sense is of most value in murky water or in revealing prey hidden close by. Some bony fish, such as catfish, have similar electric organs which are situated along the body in the canals which form part of their lateral line system.

Most fish use electricity only in a passive way, receiving the tell-tale discharges of other animals. Some, though, have adopted a more aggressive approach.

THE STUNNERS

The numbfish, which Pliny the Elder recorded in the first century AD, are now known as electric rays. The secret of their ability to paralyse animals in their vicinity lies in powerful electric organs on the head and gills which can generate a 90-volt high-amperage current. Electric rays lurk down on the ocean bed, often in shallow water,

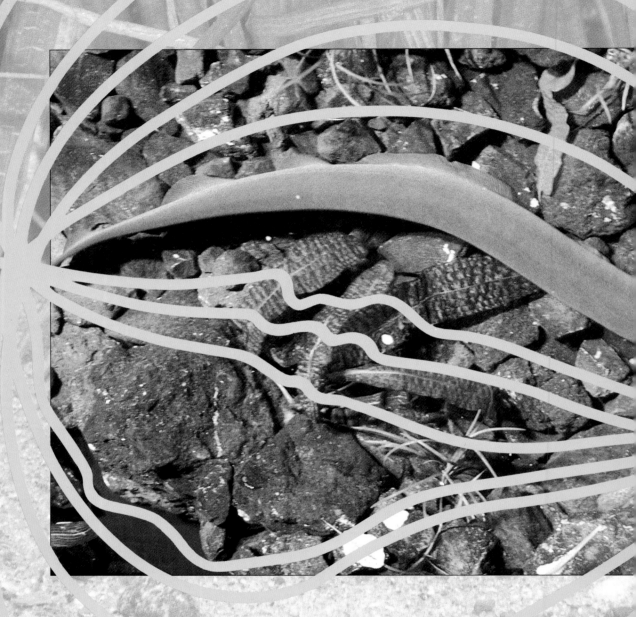

Electric fish sense their surroundings through an electric force field generated by specially modified muscle cells. As the fish swims, the field is distorted by any objects it passes. The nature of these distortions depends on how well these objects conduct electricity. In the main picture the force field is represented by the lines around the fish. Plants, which conduct electricity readily, cause the lines to converge, while rocks, which are poor conductors, cause the lines to diverge. These variations in the field are picked up by sensors along the fish's body. The illustration shows an electric eel. This fish is able to step up the voltage of the field to stun any fish that passes into it.

and they can deliver a painful shock to any person unfortunate enough to step on one. This ray does not need to move very much because its electricity does most of the work of catching food. Once its discharges have stunned prey, the electric ray simply undulates its disc-like body to create a current of water which carries the meal to its mouth.

Another kind of fish, the electric catfish, has a similar ability. Adults grow to over a metre long and generate electricity of up to 300 volts, while even baby electric catfish only 2 centimetres long can produce 10 volts. However, electric rays have a big advantage over these fish. Electric catfish live in the Nile and Congo rivers of Africa, and the fresh water of their homes is a much poorer conductor of electricity than the salt water surrounding the marine rays. As a result, the 300 volts created by the adults only has a stunning effect if the prey is very close.

The most lethal of all electric fish has solved this problem by stepping up the voltage. The tail of the electric eel contains 10 000 tiny electric organs, arranged in 70 columns, and over half of the fish is given over to electricity production. This allows it to generate an incredible 550 volts. In fact, such voltages can even kill a person.

Some of these electric fish also generate much smaller electric fields to sense their surroundings. Relatives of the electric eel, the weakly electric knife-fish of South America, and an unrelated group, the mormyrids of Africa, also use this technique.

ELECTRIC FIELD GENERATORS

The knife-fish and the mormyrids generate their electricity in columns of modified muscle cells. The output from these is not strong enough to harm other animals, rarely rising above a single volt. However, it is sufficient to produce an electric field surrounding the fish and its immediate neighbourhood. Any electric field is affected by how well objects within it conduct electricity. So, obstacles or other animals in the vicinity reveal themselves by distorting the fish's electric field. Electroreceptors along the fish's body continually monitor the field and detect any distortions to build up an electrical pattern of the surroundings. The receptors are linked to the same area of the brain as the eyes, and so the fish can probably visualise these electrical patterns, although they would only form a crude, shadowy image.

These fish do not generate electricity continuously, but switch on and off rapidly. Many do this smoothly, producing oscillating waves with a frequency of about 50 hertz – the same frequency as the mains electricity in our homes – although some can vary the rate and, depending on the species, may reach as high as 2000 hertz. Others produce much more irregular rapid click-like pulses.

All these fish use their fields to locate prey. Pulse-producing species improve the definition of their electrical picture as they home in on prey by clicking at a faster rate. Wave-producing species create a similar effect by increasing the voltage of the field.

Electric fish communicate rich and varied information to each other through their fields. An individual's field can reveal its sex, age, and emotional state, and it is also used in courtship displays. However, there is a danger that the fish's own field could block out the electrical chatter of others. Pulse-generating species emit such short and irregular clicks that they rarely jam each other and most gregarious electric fish are of this type. Wave-producing species shift their frequencies slightly to avoid confusion with nearby fish operating on the same frequency.

Another problem which electric fish have circumvented is that very sensitive receptors are needed to pick up the weak signals of other fish, and such receptors would be swamped by the fish's own field. So, the mormyrid group of electric fish have two types of receptors – highly sensitive ones for picking up messages, and less sensitive ones for monitoring their own field. The communication receptors are switched off each time a field is generated.

These fish have developed their electric sensors to perform a wide range of functions. However, they respond to other stimuli as well as electricity in order to build up a fuller picture of their environment. None of the creatures with a special sense relies on it exclusively, and many also utilise senses similar to our own. Even familiar senses can contribute towards extraordinary powers as that king of the oceans, the shark, demonstrates.

COMBINING SENSES

The film industry has made the shark one of the most feared and familiar of all fish. In reality, this much-maligned creature rarely kills people, and any attacks are usually caused by one of the shark's senses becoming confused.

A hunting shark closing in for the kill homes in on the body electricity given off by its victim. The shark may confuse the electricity of a swimmer with that of a fish, with fatal results for the human. Unfortunately, injured people give off more electricity and so are particularly vulnerable.

Such mistakes are rare, however, because the shark has a magnificent array of other senses. It can detect the minute water movements produced by the muscular twitches of its prey. The shark's hearing is remarkably sensitive, and it can even hear the sounds made by a swimming fish. Its eyes are ten times more sensitive to light than our own and, as they are tuned to the colour of the undersea world, they see a very different view from the one familiar to divers. In addition, it can locate prey by smell alone, scenting blood from well over half a kilometre away. Combined, these senses make the shark's world more remarkable than any celluloid image could possibly convey.

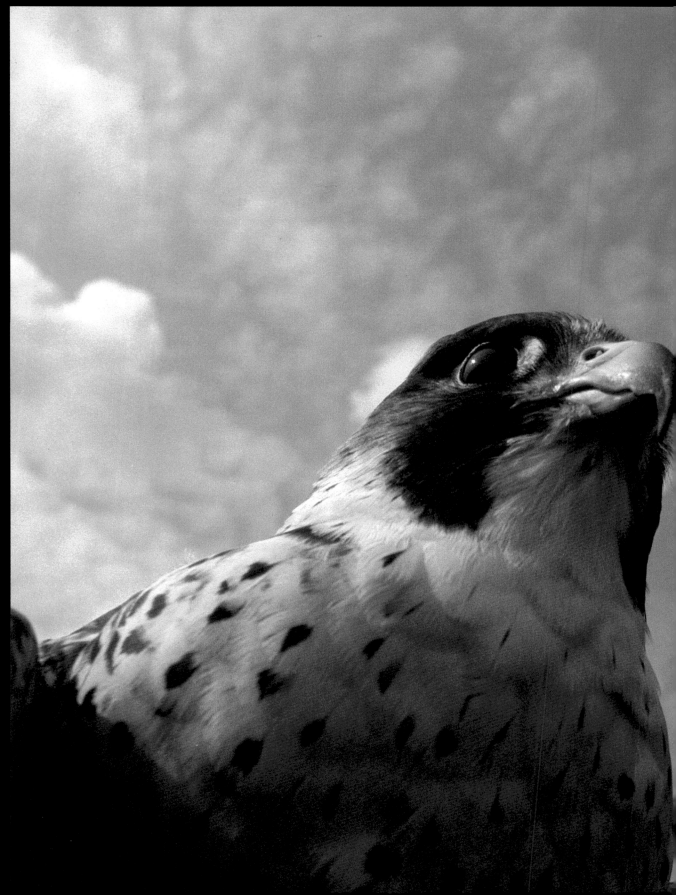

■ SEEING SENSE

We rely on light more than any other stimulus to gather information about our surroundings. As a result, our eyesight is so well developed that few animals possess comparable vision, and we are justified in considering it our supersense.

Sight is so important to us that it dominates the way we perceive the sensory worlds of other animals, and even dictates the vocabulary available to describe those worlds. When a fish depends heavily on electricity or water movements to respond to its environment, we visualise it using the stimulus to form an image or picture of its surroundings. In fact, electricity, water waves and light are all affected by surrounding objects, although in slightly different ways, and so can all be used to reveal the environment.

When we view a scene, we are gaining an impression of our surroundings by the way in which light is absorbed or reflected from objects, but light is only part of a vast spectrum of electromagnetic waves. Our eyes can detect only certain wavelengths of this spectrum, but we have built machines which can respond to other wavelengths. Electromagnetic waves with lengths ranging from several kilometres to less than a metre can be picked up by tuning a radio into long or short wavebands. Radar and some ovens make use of microwaves, which are only a few centimetres or millimetres long. Shorter wavelengths are felt by us as heat, and are also given off in the warmth of our bodies. The pit organs of snakes can gather these infra-red rays to form a crude heat picture.

The radiation which we call light covers a tiny band of the spectrum, consisting of waves about 400–700 millionths of a millimetre (400–700 nanometres) long. We are able to both detect and colour-code the different wavelengths in this band. The longer wavelengths reflected by, for example, the leaves of trees in autumn, appear to us as reds and oranges, while the shorter wavelengths which reach our eyes from the ocean we see as greens and blues.

The eyes of other animals are often sensitive to a slightly different band. Some freshwater fish can see further into the red or longer wavelength part of the spectrum than we can. At the other end of the band, many insects, fish and birds are able to see beyond blue into ultraviolet radiation invisible to us. Shorter wavelengths than this can cause damage to animal tissue and so they are not used by any life, except us. We cannot view them directly, but with the aid of machines we utilise the penetrating power of short X-rays and gamma rays to look inside the human body and diagnose illnesses.

Even the band of wavelengths that we share with other animals may create very different impressions, for there are a wide variety of eye designs in the natural world. Birds have similar eyes to ourselves, but some can enhance a portion of the field of view to create a telephoto image while others can see a far greater range of hues. Insects use a matrix of tiny lenses, and those of a dragonfly number a staggering 30 000. Other invertebrates may collect light with natural mirrors, while some crustaceans scan the scene in front of them, extracting a picture in a similar way to the moving dot in a television camera.

The design of eye is not the only feature which determines an animal's view of the world. We accept without a second's thought that we can open our eyes and observe everything around us, picking out the slightest movement. Our ability is mainly due to the brain which receives information about the brightness and wavelengths of light hitting the eyes and converts these into a multi-coloured, three-dimensional image. Such intricate processing requires a lot of brain power, and we are prepared to devote this because sight is so important to us. Other animals often depend as much or more on different senses, and allocate much less of their brain to sight. So, an animal with eyes of a similar design to ours may perceive a much less detailed image than we do.

A huge diversity of vision has arisen in the natural world because the sun is such an important influence on life. Virtually every creature is able to detect the sun's light, although some can only distinguish between light and darkness.

SENSING LIGHT

Most plants use the sun's light to manufacture their food through a process known as photosynthesis. They sense this energy using a pigment, chlorophyll, which changes form in light and so is called photo-sensitive. Animals rely on another type of photo-sensitive pigment, known as rhodopsin, to detect light.

Single-celled animals may have their pigments scattered, or gathered together to form an eye-spot in the cell. More complex animals usually devote whole cells to receiving light. Again, these may be dotted around the surface of the body or collected in one or more eye-spots. The photo-sensitive cells can detect whether it is light or dark, but give no other information.

Starfish, flatworms and other early animals use a slightly refined system in which the eye-spots are placed in a cup-like depression. The cup shadows the cell and so the animal can gain an impression of the direction of the light source. Later animals had deeper cups filled with many light-sensitive cells, until gradually more complex true eyes evolved, and made eye-spots redundant.

However, some insects have well-developed eyes and yet retain simple eyes. Those of the dragonfly are placed on either side of the head and seem to act as horizon detectors. Sensitive only to the difference between the light sky and the dark ground, and unable to distinguish distracting detail, the simple eyes are marvellous flight aids, helping the dragonfly maintain a level course. Swallowtail butterflies also retain light-sensitive cells, this time on their sexual organs. The mating of these butterflies involves joining hooks and claspers, and it is thought that the eye-spots aid this rather complicated sexual manoeuvre.

SIMPLE EYES

In the simplest true eyes, the opening of the cup-like depression is narrowed. So, the photo-sensitive cells lining it receive not just an impression of light or darkness, but a crude image of the scene. This effect was used in the very early cameras, which did not have a lens but produced an image by admitting light through a pinhole. When the opening of such a camera is large, rays of light from nearby points spread out and overlap on the screen, forming a fuzzy image. As the hole narrows, the overlap of light from nearby points decreases until eventually a reasonably clear image is obtained.

An ancient marine mollusc, known as nautilus, has an eye like a pin-hole camera. It lives in a beautiful multi-chambered shell, which provides buoyancy and protection. These animals have changed little during the 400 million years since they evolved, and still retain their strange eyes. Each eye is about a centimetre across and is packed with up to 4 million light receptors, lit through an opening which can be varied from 3 millimetres down to a tiny 0.4 millimetres. With the opening closed right down, this system could give the nautilus quite a clear picture of a brightly lit scene. However, for most of the time its underwater home is not well-lit, and the opening has to be enlarged to admit enough light.

The vital ingredient which the nautilus's eye lacks is a lens. An eye with this device can have a large opening, relying on the lens to bend the light so that spreading rays converge to form a sharp image. Many invertebrates and all vertebrates incorporate a lens in their eye.

Most spiders have eight eyes, although only two of them are sophisticated enough to create a picture of the scene. The simpler side eyes detect peripheral movement and guide the main eyes towards potential prey. Only the main, forward-facing eyes provide an image of any quality. They focus particularly on the number of legs in view – six legs indicate food, while eight suggest a potential mate. These eyes contain a lens which directs light onto photo-receptive cells arranged in layers to form a retina. The retina is unusual in that it can be moved to scan the scene. This system is quite successful, and

THE VISIBLE SPECTRUM

Only a small portion of the electromagnetic spectrum can be seen by animal eyes. This band of energy is known as light. Our eyes are able to code much of this light in terms of colour, an ability we share with closely related species such as baboons.

On either side of our visible spectrum are wavelengths that some other animals can detect. By using special pit organs, pythons and rattlesnakes can see the far-red radiation given off by living bodies. Using conventional eyes, goldfish can not only see near-infrared but also ultraviolet – both these wavelengths are invisible to our eyes. Some birds can also detect ultraviolet; and many insects have their vision shifted towards this light. Fish that live in the deep oceans have their eyes tuned only to the blue colour of the ambient light.

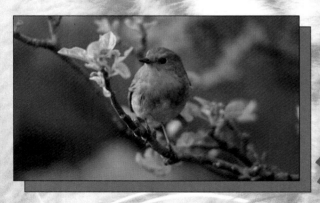

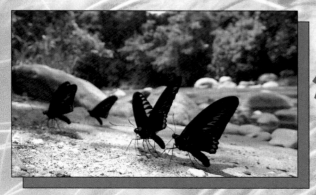

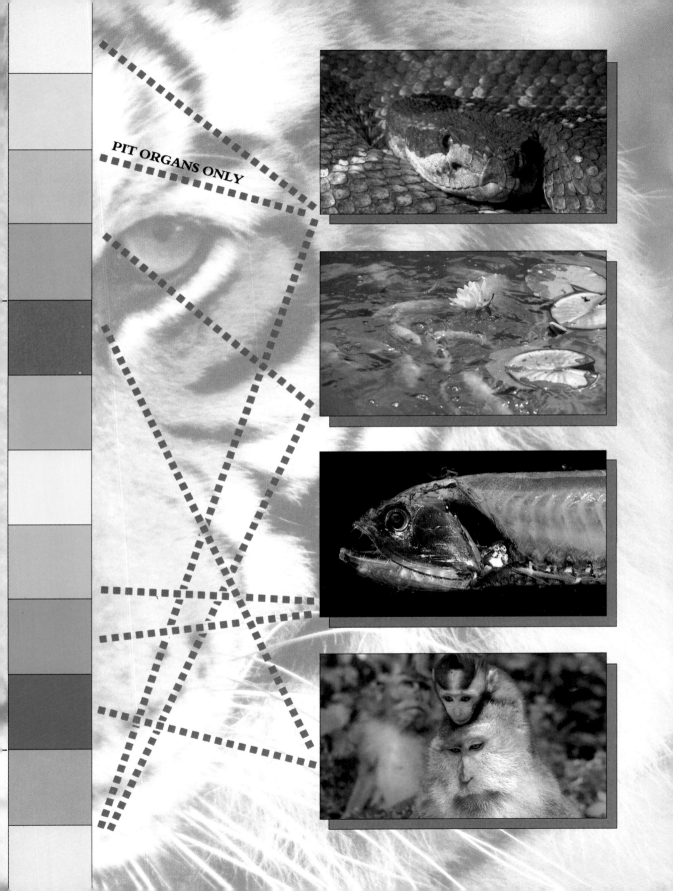

PIT ORGANS ONLY

the main eyes of the hunting spider, *Portia*, compete with those of some vertebrates, and produce an image only about six times poorer than our own eyes.

CAMERA EYES

The eyes of all vertebrates follow a similar design, which can be likened to that of a modern camera. In land animals, the transparent window at the front of the eye, the cornea, acts like the first element of a camera lens and bends or refracts the light entering the eye. This refraction occurs because light travels at a different speed in air than in the cornea. However, the speed of light is roughly the same in the cornea as in water, and so a fish's cornea simply protects the eye without bending the light.

Behind the cornea is a pigmented area known as the iris, which gives the eye its colour. The rays pass through a hole in the iris, called the pupil, which opens or closes automatically to alter the amount of light entering the eye, just as the diaphragm of a camera adjusts its aperture. Behind the iris is the curved lens, and this bends light coming from either air or water. The lens projects the light onto the retina to form an upside-down image. Fish bring the image into focus in a similar way to a camera, by moving the lens towards or away from the retina. Mammals adjust the focus by making the elastic lens bulge more, or flattening it.

The focused light hits a mosaic of rod- or cone-shaped light detectors, which make up the retina. Each rod or cone contains a photo-sensitive pigment and the changes this undergoes when exposed to light cause a signal to be passed to nerve cells at the front of the retina. The retinal nerve cells process some of the information and then send it through the optic nerve to the brain. For example, the human eye has over 130 million rods and cones, and the retina codes and combines the data so that it can be fed into the 1 million fibres entering the optic nerve.

Our brain not only turns the image the right way up, but also adds a considerable amount of detail. As you read this, only one word at a time is sharply in focus. Yet you still receive a clear impression of your surroundings, and can recognise any objects in your field of view. The brain is so good at filling in, that although most of the time the bulk of our image is blurred and lacks detail and colour, we do not realise it.

The eyes of primitive vertebrates do much more of the processing. The frog has several types of retinal nerve cells, each sensitive to different components of the picture. Some respond only to moving edges, while others are fly detectors triggered whenever anything of the right size moves into view. The frog relies on its fly detectors so much that it probably cannot see a motionless insect, and will starve rather than eat one.

Even we analyse the retinal image in terms of edge, movement and the repetition of patterns. However, the frog does not picture the flying insect as we would, because much of its visual information never even reaches its brain. Its brain does help it to recognise distasteful or painful insects, such as bees and wasps, and stops the frog reacting to those.

The relative amount of processing performed by the eye and the brain has a big impact on the visual world of all animals. The difference between the image created by our brain and that which other animals see increases in invertebrates. For many of these, the information fed into the eye triggers automatic reactions.

The exceptions to this are relatives of the nautilus, the squid and the octopus. Their eyes are very similar to ours, although, like fish, they move the lens to bring objects into focus. The retina of the octopus has up to 20 million light receptors, while the eyes of a giant squid are huge, measuring an incredible 40 centimetres across, and may be equipped with over 1000 million light detectors – nearly 100 times more than our own eyes. These cephalopods have relatively large brains and over half of each is devoted to vision. As a result, they probably see the world very much as we do, except that their image is in monochrome, not colour.

Many other invertebrates not only have much smaller brains, but have eyes of a strikingly different design to our own.

THE COMPOUND EYE

The eyes of insects are made up of tiny hexagonal units called ommatidia. Each unit acts like an eye, and contains a small lens or facet, which focuses light down a rod (known as a rhabdom) made up of layers of light detectors. The ommatidia are packed closely together to form a multi-faceted compound eye.

This design of eye reveals far less detail than a camera eye. It has been estimated, for example, that a compound eye would need to be about a metre across to match the resolution of our eyes. However, this is not a great disadvantage, for in an insect's world, significant objects tend to loom large and close. The compound eye also has advantages. Some designs allow more light to be gathered than in camera eyes. In addition, we can only bring a small area of the view into sharp focus, whereas the compound eye sees equally clearly over its whole field of vision.

There are various types of compound eyes. In that of most daytime insects, each ommatidium is optically separated from its neighbours. So each rhabdom detects only the small portion of the view which enters one facet. This does not mean that the insect sees a fragmented scene, as has been portrayed in science fiction films. The insect combines the information from all the rhabdoms to produce a picture, and its definition depends on the number of ommatidia.

The eyes of some underground worker ants have only nine facets and so form a very indistinct image. A bee has 5000 facets and would see flowers rather as they might appear in a pointillist painting. The dragonfly has so many ommatidia that it can see as

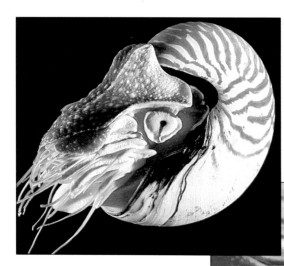

The nautilus (*left*) has no lens in its eye so its vision is poor. It can vary the opening (*centre*) to alter the amount of light reaching the light receptors. When the opening is small, objects are more sharply in focus (*see page 37*). In contrast the octopus (*below*) does have a lens and so has good vision. It focuses by moving the lens (*see page 41*).

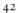

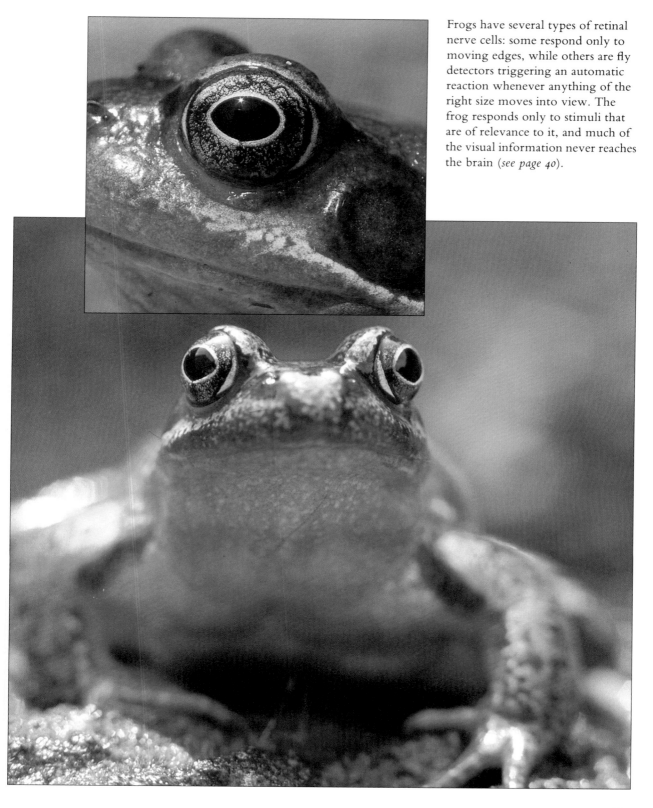

Frogs have several types of retinal nerve cells: some respond only to moving edges, while others are fly detectors triggering an automatic reaction whenever anything of the right size moves into view. The frog responds only to stimuli that are of relevance to it, and much of the visual information never reaches the brain (*see page 40*).

well as some vertebrates. Its 30 000 facets provide it with a picture rather like a grainy photograph.

Many nocturnal insects have a slightly different compound eye which allows them to gather more light. The pigments which optically separate one ommatidium from another are withdrawn at night so that each rhabdom can receive light from many facets. This slightly coarsens the image, but without this adaptation, the eye might not admit enough light to form an image at all.

Crustaceans also have compound eyes and some, such as crayfish and shrimps, have a novel variation. The eyes have square facets below each of which is a box-like chamber with mirrored sides. Light entering the facets is reflected off the mirrors down to the light detectors, creating an extremely bright image.

Some owners of compound eyes have another bonus to compensate for their poor resolution, and that is the rate at which they can perceive images.

FLICKER FUSION

If a fly strayed into a cinema, its view of the film would be very unlike that of the human audience. Its compound eye resolves less detail and so the image would look both much coarser and grainier. However, the most striking difference is that it would see not a motion picture, but a succession of still frames, rather like a slide show. This is due to the fly's much higher flicker fusion frequency.

When an image hits the retina of the eye, it lingers for a fraction of a second. If another image occurs during this time, we cannot perceive any interval between the first and second images and they appear continuous. The number of images per second needed to make them merge is called the flicker fusion frequency. In bright light we can distinguish 60 images per second. However, in poor light our rate can drop below 10, and in a cinema the 24 frames per second on the film merge into a continuous moving picture.

The light receptors of a fly restore much more quickly and its flicker fusion frequency is 300 per second. If we had such a high rate, many of our devices would become irritating or disturbing. On the television screen, we would see the moving scanner building up a picture 25 times each second. We would even detect the variation in mains electricity, which has a frequency of 50 hertz. All our electric bulbs would flicker, while fluorescent tubes would flash on and off like disco lights.

For fast-moving animals, such as flies, bees and dragonflies, however, the ability to take in many images each second is a great advantage. It helps them to follow the scene in their high-speed world, and so track the rapid movements of predators or' prey. Nocturnal insects need time to gather enough light to form an image, and so their flicker fusion frequency is quite low, that of nocturnal crickets being about 45 per second.

To most animals, the clarity of each image is at least as important as the number per second, and many have found ways of sharpening up the picture.

GETTING IN FOCUS

The cornea helps to focus the light hitting our eyes, but the fine focusing is performed by the lens. This is a mass of tightly-packed transparent sheets in an elastic case, held by muscles. Usually, the lens is only slightly rounded and focuses the distant parts of a scene. If an object is brought nearer, the muscles squeeze the lens, making it more rounded, so that it can bring the nearby object into focus. This change, called accommodation, happens automatically in people with normal eyes, and so we only become aware of the process when it starts to go wrong. People with poor accommodation, due to eye defects or age, have to wear artificial lenses to compensate.

The range of distances that animals can focus on or accommodate is measured in dioptres. We have very good accommodation compared with most other mammals. A child's range is usually about 14 dioptres, although the range decreases with age, that of an old person being only about 1 dioptre. Dogs, on the other hand, have to put up with a range of 1 dioptre all their lives. Many animals have equally poor accommodation or none at all.

Unusually, pigeons and chickens can bend their corneas as well as their lenses to help them bring objects into focus. The flying fox has a more ingenious technique. This bat feeds on fruit and uses vision to guide it from its roost to the food. Steering through foliage at night, it needs good accommodation and it achieves 5 dioptres by changing the shape of its lens and having a corrugated retina. The corrugations increase the focusing range by varying the distance between the lens and the retina.

Fish, squid and octopuses accommodate solely by moving the lens towards or away from the retina. Underwater animals have a problem in focusing because light travelling through water is not bent by the cornea, and the lens has to do all the work. Fish have overcome this difficulty by having almost spherical lenses. Artificial lenses of this shape are optically poor, but a fish's lens is designed so that it corrects these aberrations, achieving a quality of image with a single lens which camera manufacturers are still trying to match.

The lens in our eyes cannot bulge enough to focus underwater, and other swimmers appear blurred, although still recognisable as people. Inserting a layer of air, for example by wearing diving goggles, restores the clear image. Many aquatic animals have similar difficulties when they come onto land. Seals have almost spherical lenses and cannot

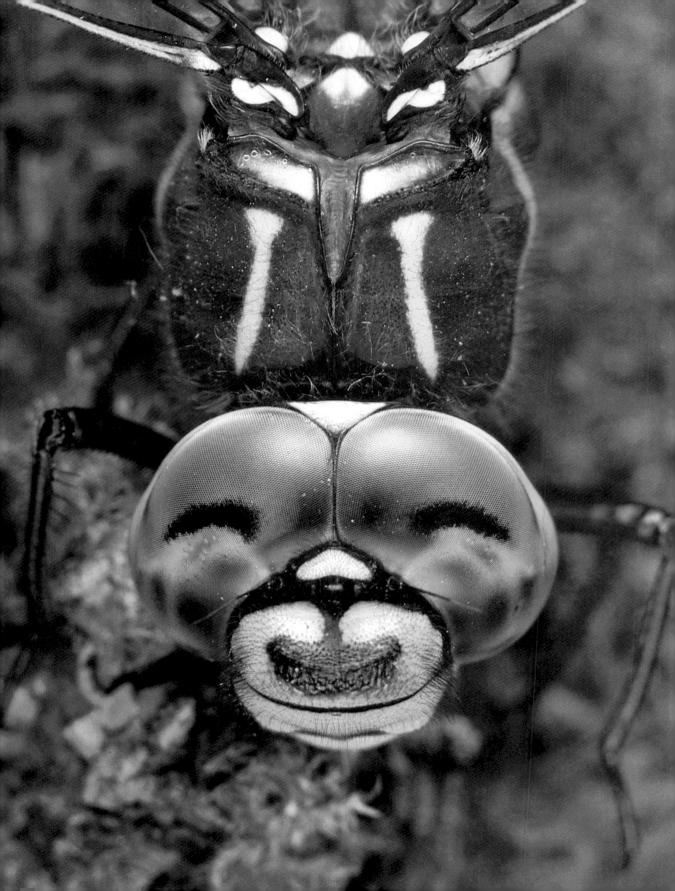

The dragonfly (*far left*) has 30 000 facets in each of its compound eyes, which allows it to see a detailed view of the world (*see page 41*). The bee (*below*) responds to ultraviolet light (*see page 57*): the celandine (*centre*) looks a uniform yellow to us, but the bee sees it as having a dark centre (*left*) and is guided towards this to find the pollen.

flatten them enough to see far through the air. However, some animals have developed eyes which can cope with the transition from air to water.

Diving birds, such as cormorants and mergansers, have additional muscles around the lens, which can drastically alter its shape and may even be able to squeeze the lens through the iris. This system gives them an accommodation of 50 dioptres, the greatest focusing range of any animal. The surface-dwelling fish, *Anableps*, has come up with a different solution – its eyes are split to create two extra eyes. As *Anableps* swims along, one pair of eyes scans the air for predators, while the other pair examines the water for food. Each air eye shares a lens with a water eye but has a separate pupil and retina. Light from the two pupils follows different paths through the oval lens, and so are brought into focus on their separate retinas.

In contrast to these animals, many invertebrates do not need to accommodate at all. Each facet of the compound eye, and each spider's eye, is so small that it has a short focal length. This gives it a great depth of field, and everything is maintained in focus.

ADDING FINE DETAIL

Only large eyes can resolve fine detail, so the tiny facets of insects' eyes and the small eyes of spiders have poor resolution. Some flies have larger facets at the front and top of the compound eye to pick out detail. The male hoverfly uses these to keep the tiny female in view as he chases her during courtship, while robberflies use them to track their flying prey.

The resolution of animals with large eyes is limited by the number of light receptors they have, and how closely these are packed together. We have 200 000 receptors per square millimetre, giving us very good resolution. However, the sparrow's eye has double this density, while the buzzard's retina contains an astounding 1 million per square millimetre.

In many animals, including ourselves, the light receptors are not spread uniformly across the retina, but are concentrated in areas known as foveae. These areas also have the greatest number of nerve connections. As you move your eyes across this page, one word at a time is focused onto the fovea. Our fovea is centrally placed and circular in shape, a characteristic we share with animals which live in forests and other visually complex environments. Animals which live in open country, such as the African bush, tend to have their fovea elongated into a strip.

Birds usually have an elongated fovea to see detail on the horizon, and most have an additional circular fovea facing straight ahead. Birds of prey, which are among the keenest-sighted animals in the world, have two circular foveae in each eye as well as a strip. Each circular fovea forms a deep concave pit, and this adaptation has a remarkable effect. The pit acts like a telephoto lens, magnifying the image which falls on the fovea and giving these birds superb vision. Vultures may rise up each morning on columns of air called thermals, reaching heights of 2000 metres or more. We cannot discern a bird at this altitude, but the vulture is able to survey the land for many kilometres around it, and locate a fresh kill. Other birds of prey perform similar feats as they hunt down live animals.

Another crucial factor in helping them locate prey is the position of their eyes.

PREDATORS AND PREY

If you look at yourself in the mirror, you are gazing into the eyes of a predator. Our eyes are placed at the front of the head, a position shared by the eyes of cats, birds of prey and other hunters. Prey animals, such as rabbits and ducks, need to observe as much of their surroundings as possible so that predators do not catch them unawares. As a result, the hunted have an eye on either side of the head.

The difference between the views of predator and prey is considerable. Many hunted animals can scan 360 degrees, giving them wrap-around vision. Without moving our heads, we can see about 208 degrees around us, while a cat's field of view is only about 187 degrees.

Predators can, of course, usually scan the entire field by moving the head, and the owl's head is so mobile that it will turn through 360 degrees. The chameleon sweeps the scene with less effort. Each eye has only a narrow field of view, but it can be swivelled independently to scan over a hemisphere. When one eye spots a potential prey, the other converges to focus on it too. Some deep-sea fish have developed another solution. They have an additional lens at the side of the eye which focuses light onto a separate retina. This increases the fish's view just as a car's rear-view mirrors give us an impression of the scene behind.

A predator's narrow field of view does have an advantage, for it increases the amount of overlap in the images received by the two eyes. A rabbit has an overlap of only 24 degrees, while we manage an amazing 180 degrees. Receiving two images of the same area allows greater detail to be picked out and improves sensitivity when the light is poor. In most animals, this binocular overlap is at the front. However, some birds, such as snipe, have eyes towards the back of the head, giving them overlap at the rear. The bittern's eyes are low down on its head, and so it can stand concealed in the reeds with its head pointing up, scanning the water below.

Perhaps the greatest value binocular vision has for us is that it allows us to judge distance. One eye alone can give clues to depth. For example, if the head is moved, the image of nearby objects shifts more than those further away. Scenes can also be given perspective by colour and shading. We are also able to detect the change in shape of the eye's lens as it focuses on an object. The chameleon can judge distances so accurately

■ FOVEAL VIEWS

■ Both the cheetah and its gazelle prey have the sharpest and most detailed parts of their vision elongated into a horizontal strip, as shown on the main picture. This is where the light receptors reach the greatest density on the retina. These animals live in the vast expanse of open savannah, and this design allows both predators and prey to keep a wide area of their field of view in focus. In comparison, we live in a complex visual environment with more vertical structures and so our foveal view, represented by the dotted circle on the main picture, need not be elongated. In both cheetah and man, the rest of the visual field shows little detail and is out of focus, but the brain fills in much of the missing information.

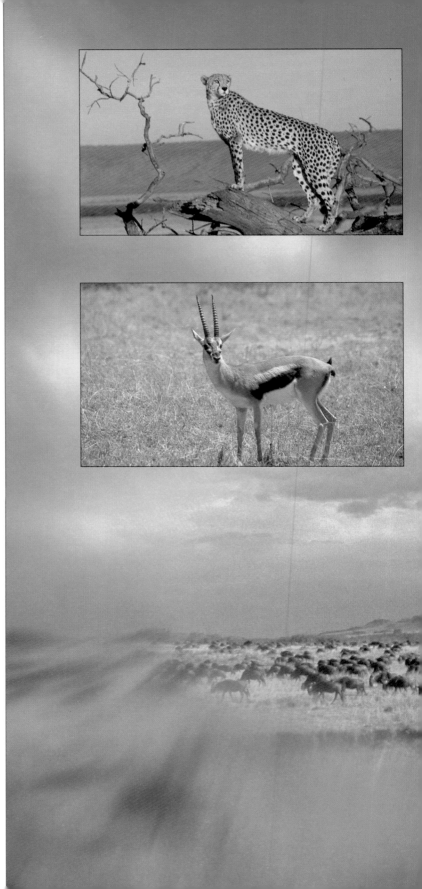

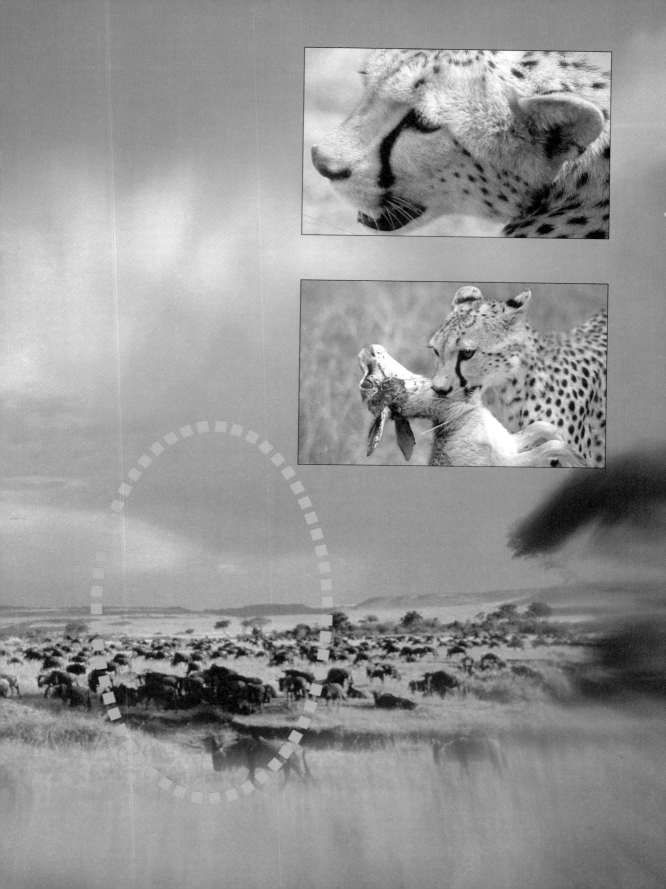

by this method that it is able to catch insects with one eye covered. However for us to match the skill of the chameleon we require two eyes, for we judge depth primarily by comparing the two overlapping views we receive. Closing one eye and then the other reveals the same scene with the position of objects shifted slightly, particularly those nearby. Our brain uses these slight differences to give the scene depth and so provide us with a three-dimensional image. This requires a large area of the brain, and so it is uncertain how many other animals use their binocular vision in this way.

Our brain also colours the image, making grass a vivid green, turning skies a brilliant blue or dull grey, and giving flowers their beautiful hues. This is a complex process, involving the separation and coding of the different wavelengths in the light which reaches us, and colour vision is by no means universal among animals.

COLOURING THE SCENE

We have two sorts of light receptors in the retina, rods and cones. Only the cones can distinguish between different wavelengths and so provide the brain with the information necessary to colour the scene. There are three kinds of cones, one sensitive mainly to blue light, one to green light, and one to yellow-green light. The fact that two of our cones are sensitive to green is thought to indicate that we once lived in tropical forests, where this area of the spectrum dominates the scene. The yellow-green cone is also sensitive to the red part of the spectrum, and so is often called the red cone. The brain receives information about red, blue and green light from the cones and mixes them to produce a multi-coloured image containing a vast range of hues.

The cones are concentrated in the fovea, and the rest of the retina has a higher proportion of rods which only provide monochrome vision. The illusion of full colour outside the central image is provided by the brain. This can be demonstrated by moving a previously unseen object into a person's field of view. The person is unable to identify the colour until the object is close to their main image area.

Other primates, such as baboons and gorillas, have the same three pigments, and so see the world very much as we do. Frogs also respond to similar colours but, again, because most of their visual information is processed by the eye itself, their view is unlikely to be anything like our own. Instead, colours produce an automatic reaction. For example, the frog is very sensitive to blue and when in danger instinctively leaps towards the nearest blue area, which in most cases is water.

Some people lack one colour pigment, and so lose sensitivity to part of the spectrum, usually red or green. They share this deficiency with squirrels, dogs and many other mammals, which naturally have only two pigments and have difficulty distinguishing between reds and greens.

It is often difficult to assess the colour vision of mammals, and some which were thought to see in monochrome have been shown to have sensitivity to colour. For example, it was said that bulls could not distinguish the red of a matador's cloak, but recent studies have shown that cattle can detect colours to a certain extent. In fact, it is likely that all mammals have some colour vision, although it is poorly developed in nocturnal animals, such as the cat. This night prowler has a low density of cones in its retina and so can only see colour in objects which fill a large part of its field of view. As the cat moves closer to an object, its colour definition improves.

There are some people whose cones are sensitive to different wavelengths than normal, giving them a unique view of the world. This is rare in humans, but among guppies variation in colour pigments is common. In fact, each guppy in a tank may see the world coloured slightly differently from its fellows. This also occurs among marmosets and squirrel monkeys. Each squirrel monkey has two or three pigments, selected from a total of five. So, the number of hues as well as the range varies from monkey to monkey.

The shanny and marine stickleback have five pigments in their eyes, allowing them to discern more hues than we can. The best-developed colour vision of any creatures, though, is that of birds. These animals not only have five pigments in their retinas but also each cone has an oil drop which filters the light, narrowing the band of wavelengths it responds to. Birds have five different filters available to combine with their five pigments, creating a powerful system for discerning subtle hues.

Each bird has the cones and filters arranged to suit its particular needs. The pigeon has red and orange oil droplets concentrated on the view ahead and below, which is normally the ground. These filters probably enhance the colour variations in green vegetation. Seabirds which hunt on the surface of the water use red oil droplets to cut out blue scattered light.

Aeroplane pilots used to wear similarly tinted glasses as haze filters. The birds' filters enhance their sensitivity to red, and this has been exploited by other creatures. Distasteful insects often have bright red or orange warning colours, while flowers pollinated by hummingbirds are coloured red to attract them. Similarly, plants reliant on birds to disperse their seeds have red fruits and berries.

However, red filters darken the sky and this is a disadvantage for aerial hunters, which need their prey silhouetted against a light sky. Swallows and house martins have dispensed with them altogether to gain a clear view of the insects they catch on the wing. Underwater predators, such as shags and razorbills, use very few red filters because the light in sea water is predominantly blue or green. Animals which live permanently underwater have eyes specially adapted to the hues of their aquatic home.

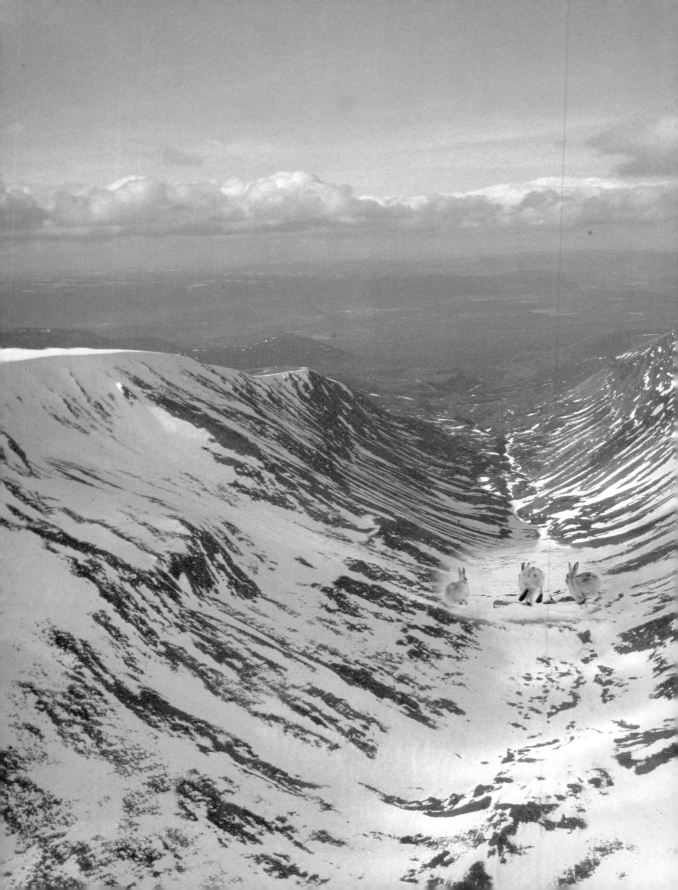

THE EAGLE'S EYE

■ The eagle's sight is legendary. Like other birds of prey, its eye provides a wide and detailed view of the world. The inner portion of its view is slightly magnified and has greater definition. The picture here is slightly exaggerated: the actual magnification is believed to be approximately ×2. The magnification is provided by an indented area of the retina which acts similarly to a lens in a telephoto system. This magnified area helps an eagle to spot Arctic hares and other camouflaged prey against a background of snow. An eagle depends on good light for its remarkable sight; in failing light our own vision is superior.

UNDERWATER COLOUR

As divers descend in the sea they experience dramatic colour changes. Orange and red light is rapidly filtered out, and only 25 metres down a red wetsuit looks almost black, while a cut at this depth oozes green blood. At greater depths, the only light piercing the abyssal gloom is a narrow band of blue. Variations of hue are indistinguishable, and many deep-sea animals make the most of the ambient light by tuning all their visual pigments to blue. Even shallow water animals with colour vision, such as penguins and elephant seals, show most sensitivity to blue light.

In fresh water, the colour bias may be very different. Rivers and lakes are often coloured green by algae or brown by decaying plants, and many freshwater fish show a peak of sensitivity to red light. This change in hues is most problematic for fish, such as salmon and eels, which migrate between fresh and salt water. The small eyes of the immature eel employ both red and blue pigments to survey its freshwater home. To equip this fish for its incredible journey across thousands of kilometres of ocean to its spawning grounds in the Sargasso Sea, the eel's eyes grow larger and their red pigments are replaced by a second type of blue pigments. Similarly, when the salmon returns to fresh water to spawn, a proportion of its pigments switch from blue-sensitive to red-sensitive.

The red shift of some freshwater fish is so extreme that they can see light invisible to our eyes.

FAR-RED VISION

The ferocity of the piranha fish has made it famous throughout the world. Its powerful jaws equipped with razor-sharp teeth tear chunks of flesh off other fish, and shoals of piranha are reputedly able to strip even large animals, such as cattle or people, to the bone within minutes. Much less well-known but equally exceptional is this fish's ability to see longer wavelength radiation than we or most other animals can. The South American rivers where the piranha lives appear completely black to us because most of the light is absorbed by molecules of decaying vegetation dissolved in the water. These dark red molecules do not absorb far-red light, however, and the piranha's far-red shifted vision allows its eyes to pierce the gloom.

Many people share their homes with an animal which has similar powers. Like the piranha, the goldfish's natural home is water coloured red by the decay of vegetation. If human eyes were sensitive to the same radiation as the goldfish's retina, we would see the infra-red remote-control beams that operate televisions and videos. A burglar would be able to avoid the trip beam of an intruder alarm system, and a factory or office would appear illuminated by the infra-red light used by security cameras.

The goldfish can not only spy on the far-red secrets of our world, but its vision extends through the spectrum to shorter wavelength ultraviolet radiation, making it receptive to a wider band of light than almost any other animal. Our retina is sensitive to ultraviolet radiation, but the eye filters it out before it reaches the light detectors, so we miss out on much of the visual information available to other animals. Ultraviolet light is so important to insects that they use it as a main component of their colour vision.

THE WORLD OF ULTRAVIOLET

Like us, the bee has three different colour pigments but these respond to ultraviolet, blue and green, instead of blue, green and red as in our eyes. If the sensitivity of our pigments suddenly shifted over to that of the bee's, the sky would still be reassuringly blue with fluffy white clouds, while nearly everything else would take on a bizarre hue. Previously green plants would be transformed into a bewildering array of colours. The grass might appear red, some trees would become magenta, and against a light background red flowers, such as poppies, would stand out as black blooms. Flowers would not only change in colour but also reveal previously invisible patterns. For example, the lesser celandine, which usually looks a uniform yellow, would develop a dark centre.

Many other insects have a shift in colour vision similar to the bee's, and flowers have evolved to be attractive to their eyes. Ultraviolet marks on the flowers guide insects to the nectar and pollen at the centre. Some plants use these marks to dupe insects. We see a striking difference between the red helliborine orchid and the blue bellflower. To the bee's eyes, unable to detect red, their colours appear very similar and their ultraviolet markings are identical. So the bee pollinates the orchid, mistaking it for the nectar-producing bellflower.

The difference in sensitivity to red of vertebrates and insects is exploited by some crab spiders. These animals can change their colour to match the petals of flowers on which they sit, waiting to ambush insects. Their camouflage appears to be destroyed by two bright red spots, indicating to birds that these spiders are noxious. However, insects cannot see the warning spots, and to them the spider's disguise is deadly perfect.

Several fish and many birds can detect ultraviolet light, and it probably helps them to navigate. When the sun is hidden by mist or cloud, ultraviolet light pierces the haze and so reveals the sun's position. Many animals also use polarised light to find their way.

THE GUIDING LIGHT OF POLARISATION

Most light vibrates in all planes about its direction of travel. However, as the sun's rays pass through the Earth's atmosphere, some of the light is changed or polarised so that

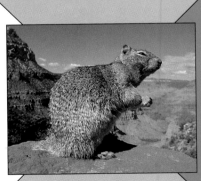

By looking at the position of animal's eyes, it is immediately apparent if an animal is predator or prey. Prey animals have their eyes positioned to the side, for they need to scan as much of the world as possible to spot approaching danger. Predators have forward-facing eyes; although this restricts their field of view, the overlap between the two views increases definition and helps with the perception of depth.

In the pictures, the light blue areas represent the fields of view that surround each animal, while the dark blue areas indicate the amount of overlap seen by the eyes.

■ A duck's 360° vision allows it to spot predators approaching from behind. As it feeds by dabbling with its bill, the small overlap between the fields of view is not a disadvantage when looking for food.

■ A squirrel is also a prey animal so it, too, needs a wide field of view. However, as it manipulates food in its paws a good overlap between the two eyes is also necessary.

Both ourselves and monkeys have a good visual overlap. Although this forward-facing vision limits the field of view, it allows depth to be judged accurately.

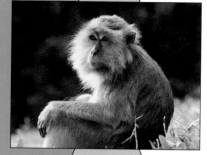

Tigers have the typical eyes of a hunter. Although they have a limited field of view, they have little to fear from other predators. The forward-facing vision allows both eyes to concentrate on their prey.

A chameleon is often hunted as well as being a hunter. Each eye has only a narrow field of view but can be swivelled independently, allowing the chameleon to see all round itself. They can even be brought together to create a visual overlap.

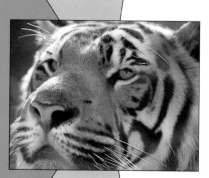

it vibrates in only one plane. The polarised light forms a pattern in the sky, which moves round with the sun and so indicates the sun's position.

Bees navigate using the sun, and for millions of years they have used polarised light to locate their guide on cloudy days. The bee detects the pattern of polarised light through special ommatidia, which occur in small regions at the top of its eyes. Even if only a tiny portion of blue sky is visible, the bee can compare this section of pattern with a reference map of the entire pattern in its brain, and pinpoint the sun.

A thousand years ago, humans used a similar but much cruder system which relied on the strongest part of the pattern, a band of polarised light arcing the sky. The Vikings took a seemingly magical crystal, known as sunstone, on their voyages. This crystal lets polarised light through only when held at certain angles. By rotating it until it cut out the polarised light, the Vikings could locate the dark polarised band.

Today we use polarised sunglasses to cut out the dazzle of polarised light reflected from water and other bright surfaces. Water striders and pondskaters, which hunt on the surface of the water, have their eyes polarised in a similar way to reduce the glare in their aquatic home. The water boatman, on the other hand, has receptors in the lower part of its eye tuned to polarised light. As it flies along, the enhanced shimmer of water helps it to find new pools. We can produce a similar effect by looking through polarised sunglasses which are turned on their side.

Uniquely, the huge eye of the squid combines these two techniques. Some of its light detectors are tuned to light polarised in one direction, while the rest are tuned to the opposite direction. Exactly what the squid sees with this strange design of eye is uncertain, but it can undoubtedly perceive great detail in highly reflective surfaces. Many fish rely on the reflection of light from their mirror-like scales to hide them, and it is likely that the squid's eye can penetrate this disguise.

Squid also inhabit deep water where the problem is not reflected light but the absence of light. Nocturnal animals have to cope with the same difficulty, and many creatures have developed ways of gathering the maximum amount of light.

SEEING IN THE DARK

When using a camera at dusk, a photographer selects the lens with the smallest f-number. This is a measure of how much light will reach the film and depends on the diameter of the lens and its distance from the film or, in the case of our eyes, the retina. The f-number of our eyes is about 2.55, while a standard camera lens has an f-number of 1.8 and special lenses may reach 1.1. No human lens, natural or artificial, can match the eye of the net-catching spider, which has an f-number of 0.58, making it 19 times more sensitive than our eyes. This Australian spider uses its remarkable night vision to throw a net-like web over its prey, rather like a miniature gladiator. The most sensitive eyes of all belong to a deep-sea crustacean called *Gigantocypris*, which manages an incredible f-0.25.

Although no vertebrate can equal their sensitivity, the eyes of the spider and crustacean are only small, and this limits the quality of their vision. For optimum clarity at night, the eyes also need to be large. The cat has relatively large eyes, and their design makes them eight times more sensitive than our own, giving it superb nocturnal vision. The eyes of a small nocturnal primate, the tarsier, are so enormous they fill most of its head. The bushbaby and barn owl also have big eyes, and, like the tarsier, their eyes are no longer spherical but swell out at the back to make the most of the available space. This means that the eyes can no longer be moved in their sockets, and these animals have developed mobile heads to compensate.

The eyes of a toad are eight times more sensitive to light than our own. Like all cold-blooded animals its night vision improves as it gets colder. This is because at low light levels, heat affects the pigment cells as much as light. So on a cold dark night the body heat of warm-blooded animals interferes with the clarity of vision, but the eyes of a toad can still pierce the gloom.

Eyes adapted for nocturnal vision are so sensitive that they need to be protected from light during the day. Some have pigment cells which move across the light detectors during the day, shielding them. Others close the pupil right down, and because of the muscular effort needed to create a small round opening, cats, crocodiles and many other nocturnal animals have pupils which close to form slits.

During the day, the centre of our field of view is clearer, but at night the peripheral view is better. This is because night vision relies mainly on the monochrome rods instead of the centrally placed colour-coded cones. The rods are able to increase sensitivity by pooling the signals from several rods before passing the information to the brain. We share this system with other vertebrates, and all nocturnal animals see mainly in monochrome. Many have another trick to make the most of the available light.

If a person shines a torch into the African bush, ghostly lights gleam back at them. There may be only a few, or they may twinkle in their hundreds like some strange city skyline and, most disconcerting of all, a double set of lights may suddenly float up and down like a luminescent yo-yo. This eerie light show is produced by the eyes of nocturnal mammals. The light from the torch hits a special reflective layer behind the retina, known as the tapetum, and some of it bounces back out again. By reflecting the light, the tapetum gives the rods a second chance to absorb the rays.

The pigments in the retina affect the colour of the reflected light, so a gazelle's eyes emit green light, a cat's eyes appear golden, while rabbits' eyes glow bright red. The tapetum is so useful for seeing in the dark that some reptiles, moths and deep-sea fish also have one. Another marine creature, the scallop, uses mirrors in one of the strangest eye designs in the natural world.

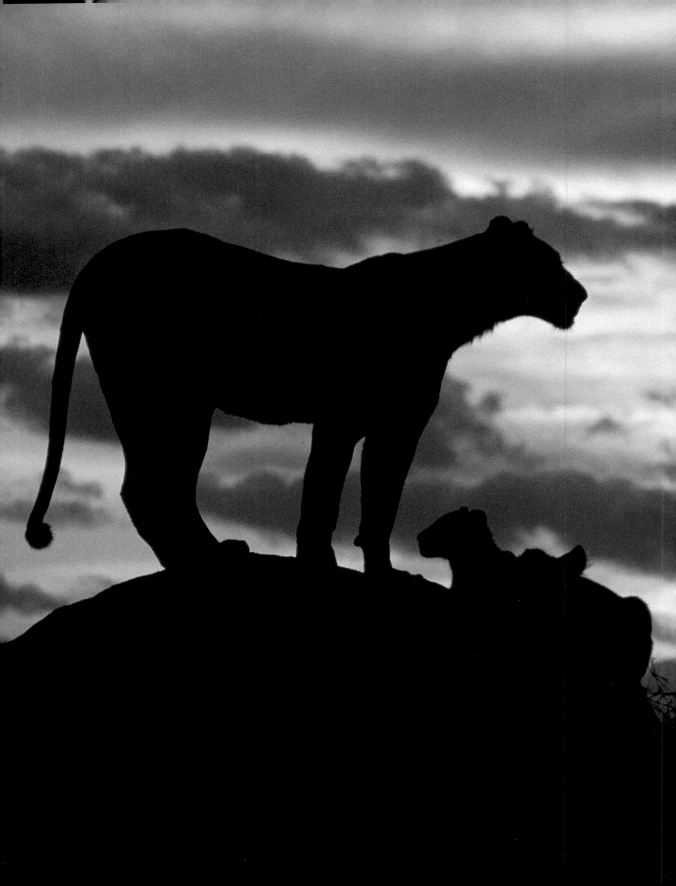

The eyes of members of the cat family are particularly well adapted for nocturnal vision: light hits a special reflective layer behind the retina, known as the tapetum, and some of it bounces out again. This reflection gives the animal's eyes a second chance to absorb the rays of light.

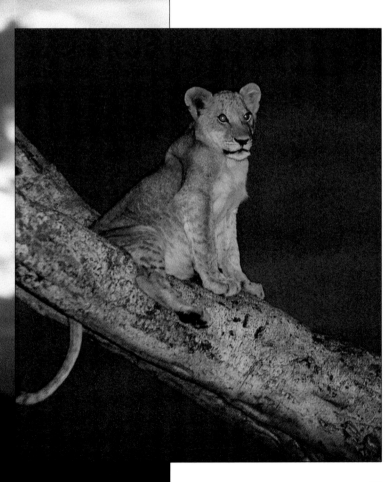

UNUSUAL EYES

If you peered into the hundred eyes of a scallop, a hundred upside-down views of yourself would peer back. The scallop has a tiny biological mirror at the back of each eye which acts as a concave reflector, focusing an image onto a retina containing 5000 light detectors. This unusual system would give the scallop superb eyesight, were it not for a design fault. The unfocused light has to pass through the retina on its journey to the mirror and this degrades the quality of the image. The scallop therefore uses its eyes to detect movement and gross variations in light and shade.

The crustacean, *Gigantocypris*, has developed a completely different design of mirror-eye. It surveys its gloomy world with two parabolic reflectors which direct light onto a retina at their centre containing nearly 1000 light detectors. Again, this design gives it only vague impressions of light and shade, but it allows the ostracod to collect a phenomenal amount of the illumination available in its dimly lit environment.

Another crustacean, *Copilia*, has perhaps the strangest eye of all, for it scans the world in a way very reminiscent of a television camera. In the camera, the image formed by the lens is scanned electronically 25 times every second. The image formed by the lens in *Copilia*'s eye is similarly scanned by a mobile second lens and retina. The retina contains only nine light detectors, but by scanning the image up to ten times each second it is able to build up some kind of picture. Another small crustacean called *Labidocera* also scans the image. Its retina forms a cup around a spherical lens, and it sees by moving the light-sensitive cup beneath the lens.

The mantis shrimp surveys its world through a unique type of compound eye. Each multi-faceted eye has a central horizontal strip consisting of rhabdoms sensitive to both colour and polarisation. Complex eye movements sweep this band across its field of view. Once it has analysed and identified potential prey, the mantis shrimp then attacks, using its club-like fore-limbs. These can deliver a punch that can reach the impact velocity of a .22 calibre bullet.

Although these animals' eyes are bizarrely constructed, they are tuned into the same light as most of the rest of the natural world. The most unusual vision of all belongs to those animals which use not only sunlight but also the light they manufacture naturally.

NATURAL LIGHT

Many people will have seen fireflies, glow-worms and other insects which create light to attract a mate during the night. This bioluminescence is more common in the oceans, where the sun's light penetrates only a few hundreds of metres down, leaving many animals in perpetual twilight or night. Many fish, squid, octopuses, comb-jellies and jellyfish ensure that the abyssal depths are never completely dark by filling them with the sparkle and shimmer of animal light. This is produced by an enzyme system which gives off light when exposed to oxygen and is a vastly more efficient process than that used by us to create artificial light. Only 10 per cent of the energy in a light bulb goes into creating light, the rest being lost as heat, while 90 per cent of bioluminescent energy is converted into light.

The viper fish and the hatchet fish have lights on their underside. They adjust the intensities of these so that they exactly match the light from the surface, making the fish effectively invisible from below.

The deep-sea angler fish uses light to catch prey. It dangles a luminous lure on the end of a rod sticking out from its head, and any animals attracted by the bait are engulfed in its huge mouth.

Another fish, called Pachystomias, has evolved an even more ingenious hunting method. Long before humans devised the sniperscope, this strange fish was using a similar surveillance system. Sniperscopes rely on infra-red radiation, invisible to the human eye, to detect the enemy. Pachystomias produces a red beam, which is just as effective. Its deep-sea prey have their eyes tuned to the blue ambient light, but Pachystomias has red-sensitive pigments. So it can observe the animals illuminated by its red searchlight, while they swim in the dark, quite unaware that they are being eyed up as a potential meal.

Just as Pachystomias uses light waves invisible to its prey, many animals rely on sound waves to sense their surroundings, using wavelengths that others cannot hear. Our ears are sensitive to only a fraction of these sounds.

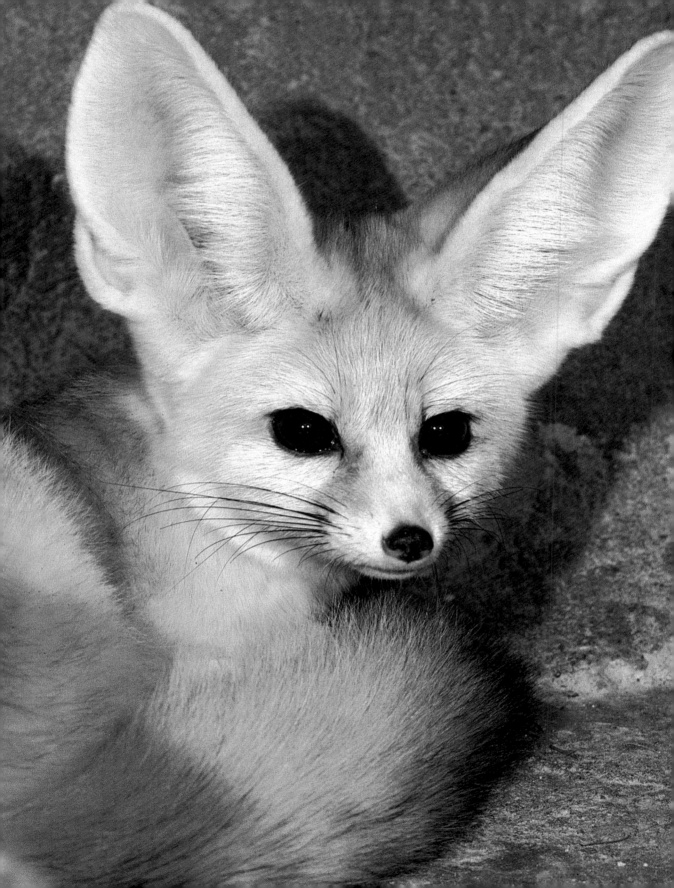

■ SOUND SENSE

Every moment vast numbers of minute air pressure waves reach our ears, most of them created by people and their machines. Our ears and brain can convert these waves into recognisable sounds – the whine of a jet plane, the rumble of traffic, the hum or clank of machinery, the ticking of a clock, the shouts or whispers of people. We can distinguish between very similar sounds, such as the ringing of an alarm, a doorbell and a telephone, and can accurately locate the sources of these sounds. If someone speaks to us, another ability is revealed for we are better at discriminating subtle changes in frequency and loudness than many other species, allowing us to use sound for complex communications.

Despite these powers, in many ways our hearing is inferior to that of many other animals. The barn owl can swoop down on a mouse in total darkness, guided only by a faint rustle in the undergrowth. As a rattlesnake strikes, the kangaroo rat leaps to safety, warned of the danger by the sound of the snake's moving scales.

Many land animals use sound to call to each other, for example, to warn of danger or to find mates. We hear only a fraction of this animal chatter. Young mice communicate in high-pitched squeaks, safe from human eavesdroppers, and spiders listen for the sound of insect wings. Away from the human-made cacophony of towns and cities, elephants call to each other through kilometres of dense forest using sounds too low for us to hear.

Underwater, we are at even more of a disadvantage, for our ears are best suited to receive air-borne sound. Here, the grunts, purrs, croaks and drums of courting fish mingle with the snapping of shrimps and the crackling of barnacles. Some whales sing duets that may last for days and show regional dialects, while others can hear calls from hundreds of kilometres away. The harmony of these underwater choirs is broken by predatory fish, which hunt by listening for their prey, and can even hear the sounds made by a swimming fish.

Most remarkable of all are the animals which detect the echoes of the sounds they create. Some use such a sophisticated system that they build up a detailed picture of their surroundings, effectively 'seeing' with sound instead of light.

This extraordinary diversity in powers of hearing is due to the different designs of ears in the natural world, and the amount of each animal's nervous system or brain which is devoted to receiving the sounds.

THE HUMAN EAR

We can get an idea of how we hear sounds by considering what happens when one person speaks to another. The speaker's vocal cords vibrate, making the molecules of air around the chords vibrate as well. The air is compressed at the same frequency as the vibrations and then expands, compressing the air next to it. In this way, the compressions or sound waves pass through the throat and mouth and out through the lips, spreading in all directions.

Some of these sound waves reach the ears of the listener and travel down each earhole to press on the stretched membrane of the eardrum. This vibrates, again at the same frequency as the vocal cords, and the vibrations pass along three bones, which span the middle ear like an arch, to another membrane called the oval window. These bones amplify the sound eighteen times, mainly because they concentrate all the waves which reach the eardrum onto the much smaller oval window. Behind this lies a fluid–filled tube, called the cochlea. Its inside surface is covered with cells which convert the sound waves into nervous impulses that the listener's brain can understand.

Any vibration which makes the surrounding molecules of air vibrate can cause sound. A large vibration creates a strong wave which we hear as a loud noise, while a small vibration produces a faint sound.

All mammals have ears which follow the same basic plan as ours. However, there are modifications to suit each animal's particular needs, which affect how the animal hears the world.

THE SOUNDS OF THE DESERT

Desert areas have little vegetation to provide shade from the heat of the sun or cover from predators. So many animals, such as the kangaroo rat, only forage during the cool of the night. In this dark, silent world, acute hearing is essential for survival.

If an owl swoops down on the kangaroo rat, the kangaroo rat is alerted by the sound of wind passing over the bird's wings and can evade the grasping talons. The rattlesnake is a more formidable enemy, because it has infra–red detectors to see in the dark and makes virtually no noise as it glides along. But the kangaroo rat can hear the faint rustles of the rattlesnake's scales moving over the sand, and escape. Even if the rattlesnake waits in ambush, it still does not succeed. In the split second of the strike, the kangaroo rat senses the sound of the moving scales and leaps to safety.

One of the reasons for its phenomenal hearing is that the kangaroo rat's eardrum is exceptionally large. The middle ear chamber is also large, probably to allow the drum to vibrate freely. In contrast, the oval window is tiny. The huge difference in size between the drum and oval window means that sounds, particularly low frequencies, are amplified 100 times, instead of just eighteen times as in the human ear.

Other animals, for example gerbils and jerboas, have similar refinements. The extreme sensitivity they gain is invaluable in their quiet desert home. In most other environments, however, such acute ears would be a disadvantage for their owners would be deafened.

GATHERING SOUND

Perhaps the most striking feature of many desert animals, such as the fennec fox and jerboa, is the size of their external ears or pinnae. These are filled with blood vessels and so help cool the animal, but they also collect and funnel sound into the earhole. The long silky ears of rabbits and hares perform the same function, and even the smaller pinnae of goats and deer are effective sound gatherers. All of these animals carry their pinnae side by side on top of the head. The pinnae usually face forward but can be swivelled round to concentrate any sound which might signal danger or food.

In comparison, our pinnae – the fleshy shells on either side of our head, which we call our ears – are poor sound gatherers. They are fairly small, usually flat against the head, and far from being able to swivel or cock them, we can barely move them. However, their strange position does allow us to locate the source of a sound.

LOCATING SOUND

At a party, our ears are being continually bombarded by the minute pressure waves generated by voices and music. Yet we can pick out and concentrate on the voice of a newcomer, or any other event which interests us, while our brain reduces the rest to a background noise. Even more surprisingly, if a glass is dropped, we can immediately turn to the source of the sound, locating its position with extreme precision.

These powers are due to the fact that we have two ears, separated by about 20 centimetres of acoustically dead grey matter. A sound to our left reaches the left ear before the right one. The time difference is tiny – less than a thousandth of a second – but the brain can not only detect this difference but also use it to compute the position of the sound source. Another clue is provided by the head blocking off waves, effectively shadowing the right ear, so that the sound reaching it is quieter. To locate faint sounds we automatically maximise the difference in time of arrival and loudness of the sound by turning our head until one ear is facing the source of the sound. Using such techniques, we can determine the direction of a noise more accurately than any other animal, with a few notable exceptions, including the barn owl.

A barn owl works out whether a sound is coming from the right or the left in the same way as we do. However, it can also tell the height of the source. It is able to do this because one of its earholes is slightly higher than the other. This difference is emphasised by the distinctive ruff on its heart-shaped face. The ruff is formed from two

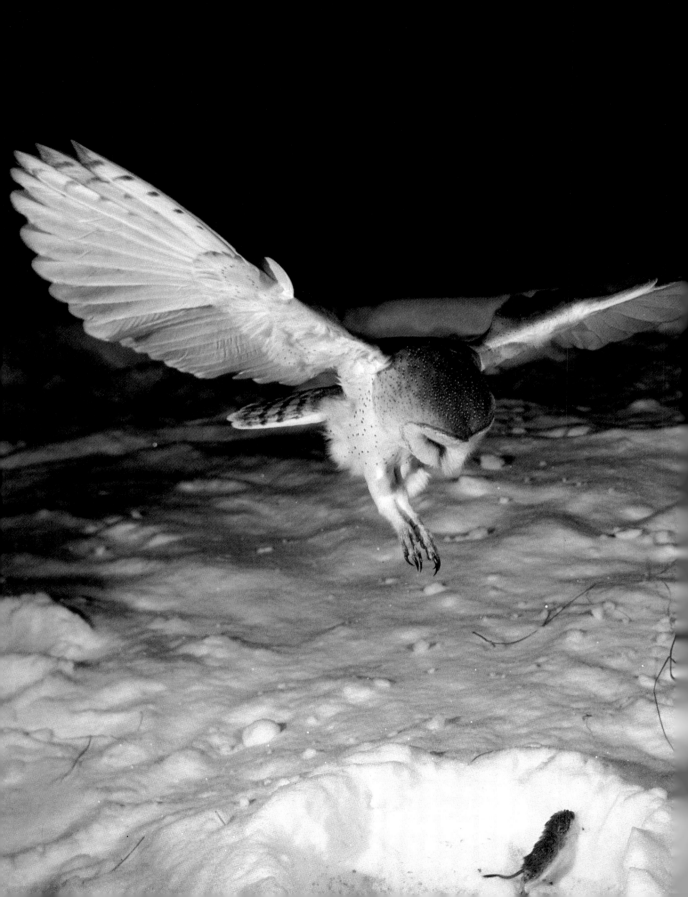

channels of tightly packed feathers, which funnel sound into the earhole. The channel on the right tilts upwards, collecting sound from above, while that on the left tilts downwards, emphasising sounds emanating below eye level. This has the effect of slightly shielding the right ear from noises emanating above eye level, while sources below eye level sound fainter to the left ear. Only a noise directly ahead at eye level sounds the same to both ears.

The barn owl's ability to locate a sound in two planes at once means that it can accurately pinpoint its prey. A large part of its brain is devoted to doing just that, and gives the owl a 'sound map' of the area around it. This system is so sophisticated that the owl can locate and memorise the position of a rustle without even moving its head and, as it swoops, it can align its claws along a mouse's body guided only by sound.

RESPONDING TO SOUND

The barn owl can not only hear and locate noises, but can also detect whether they are made by mice or other prey. Similarly, we can identify sounds with our eyes closed, even distinguishing between those which are very alike. The brain does this by recognising the rhythm and pattern of the sounds, including their frequencies.

The frequency of a sound is the number of times the air around the source vibrates each second. A slow vibration creates low-frequency waves which we hear as a low-pitched noise, while a fast vibration produces a high-pitched noise. The frequency of a sound is measured in cycles per second or hertz.

We do not respond to all frequencies of vibration. In fact, we ignore the majority of sounds present in the world. When a juggernaut passes, we only hear the rumble down to about 20 hertz, although we may feel lower vibrations. At the other end of the scale, we are deaf to some of the frequencies given off by jangling keys or screeching brakes, cutting off at around 20 000 hertz. This range of hearing does vary from person to person. Young children often hear sounds much higher than 20 000 hertz, while many 60-year-olds can only hear sounds up to 8000 hertz.

The range of frequencies that we can respond to may be partly determined by our size. Generally, large animals hear lower frequencies and small ones respond to higher frequencies. So, elephants can hear far lower sounds than us, while mice cut off below 1000 hertz but can hear sounds as high as 100 000 hertz. However, there are many exceptions to this rule because animals need to tune into the frequencies important for their survival. For example, the small kangaroo rat is very sensitive to the low-pitched sounds made by its predators and the drumming sounds made by other kangaroo rats.

Our band of hearing includes all the sounds which are significant for us – and many unwanted ones. Being deaf to all other frequencies saves our brain the work of receiving and decoding more unnecessary noises. Animals with much simpler ears and brains than us can reduce the problem further by only responding to very narrow frequency bands.

THE FINE TUNING OF FROGS

The world would sound very strange to us through the ears of a frog, for we would hear the calls of other frogs, the noises made by its predators, and little else. Its ears are only sensitive to the frequencies of these sounds and its brain will only respond to certain patterns of sound, so nearly all unnecessary noises are excluded.

To a female frog, one of the most important sounds is the mating call of the male. Her ears are so finely tuned to this that she can pick out a prospective mate's voice from a cacophony of croaks. In New Jersey, the American cricket frog's voice resounds at a frequency of 3500 hertz, and the female responds immediately to this sound. Cricket frogs in South Dakota, however, produce a call at 2900 hertz, and the females there are tuned to this deeper croak. If a female is taken from one area to the other, she ignores the local males because she is deaf to their calls.

The Puerto Rican coqui frogs use a slightly more complicated system, in which the males and females are sensitive to different frequencies. These frogs are so-named because the male's call sounds like 'ko-kee' to us, but each frog only hears one syllable. The 'ko' part announces ownership of a territory and is emitted at a frequency which other males can hear. The 'kee' part is a courtship call at another frequency which only the females are sensitive to. Like many other frogs, both sexes also respond to a band of lower frequencies. This probably allows them to detect the noise of predators.

Another amphibian, the spadefoot toad, appears to put its low-frequency hearing to a novel use. It lives in the desert and, during the long dry season, it lies dormant in a burrow under the soil. As soon as the rains come it needs to emerge quickly in order to find food, and water in which to breed. The signal for it to emerge seems to be the low-frequency noise of rain.

Equally bizarre is the sound world of many amphibians' favourite prey – the insects.

LISTENING TO WINGS

Anyone who has listened to the incessant calling of cicadas or the chirping of crickets will not be surprised to learn that insects are sensitive to sound. However, an examination of their heads will reveal no trace of an ear. In fact, crickets and cicadas hear through stretched membranes rather like our own eardrums, but these are placed in what seem to us rather odd positions. Crickets' ears are on the 'knees' of their front walking legs, while cicadas carry their ears on their bellies.

Although these insects' hearing organs are rather like our eardrums, they do not necessarily respond to sound in the same way. Our eardrum is effectively sealed and so sound waves can only reach the front part of the membrane. In many insects, the pressure waves can travel through air channels or through the tissue of the insect to vibrate the back of the stretched membrane as well. Other insects hear through clumps of hairs or special antennae which work by detecting the movement of the vibrating air molecules instead of picking up the pressure waves of sound.

As well as employing some unfamiliar ear designs, many insects tune in to frequencies which we cannot hear. Cicadas have a similar range to ourselves, hearing from 100 hertz up to 15 000 hertz. However, short-horned grasshoppers can hear sounds up to 50 000 hertz, while noctuid moths have an incredible range, from 1000 hertz up to 240 000 hertz. Within its band, each insect is particularly sensitive to the frequencies of sounds which are significant in its life, and in many cases these are the sounds of wings.

Male crickets make a noise by rubbing their wings together. One wing has a serrated surface like a file, and the other has a sharp edge over which the file is scraped. When these vibrations reach the female, she goes towards the male. As she moves, the ears on her legs keep her oriented in the direction of the call. We hear these complex vibrations as a high-pitched chirp, but to the female they sound very different. She is less sensitive to the frequency or pitch of the sound than to the timing of the pulses of sound and the variations in their loudness. Many insects respond to sound in the same way.

However some insects, such as mole crickets, are extremely sensitive to the frequency of the sound produced by their mate's wings. To ensure that its courtship sounds are heard, the male mole cricket builds an amplifier which works in a similar way to the horn of an old gramophone. It burrows into the soil and hollows out a sound chamber at the base of the burrow. The cricket periodically tests the size of its acoustic horn and adjusts it until it resonates at the frequency produced by its wings – a remarkable feat since it can only gauge the efficiency of its amplifier by detecting the changes in pressure waves within the chamber. Both the amplifier and the females' ears are tuned to the roughly 3000 hertz frequency sounds created by the male.

Female mosquitoes produce their courtship call simply by beating their wings. This was first suspected in 1878, when a row of electric lights was put up at a hotel in New York. The lights attracted male mosquitoes, which mistook the humming of the newly installed transformer for the sound of the female's wings. Away from machines, such mistakes are rare because the mosquito's system has a number of safeguards. The mating hum of the female is at a frequency of about 500 hertz and she only produces sounds at this pitch when she is ready to mate. The male, which senses her hum through his long feathered antennae, does not unfurl his wings until he is sexually mature. Once unfurled, his wings beat faster than the female's and so produce a higher hum.

Many insects communicate through wingbeats, some even using them to create special courtship songs. There are about 2000 species of fruit flies, most of which look remarkably similar. Yet they manage to avoid interbreeding, because each species has

HEARING RANGES

We hear only a fraction of the sounds that reach our ears. Animals such as foxes hear a similar range of sounds to us but can also hear many higher frequency sounds. Some animals such as frogs have their hearing tuned to very narrow frequency bands. Other have extended hearing ranges and can hear sounds that we cannot detect. Birds such as pigeons can hear the low-frequency sounds known as infrasound; elephants share this ability and use these sounds for communication. Mice and bats can hear the high-frequency sounds known as ultrasound, and use them either for communication or for echolocation. As a general rule, smaller animals hear higher frequencies than larger animals.

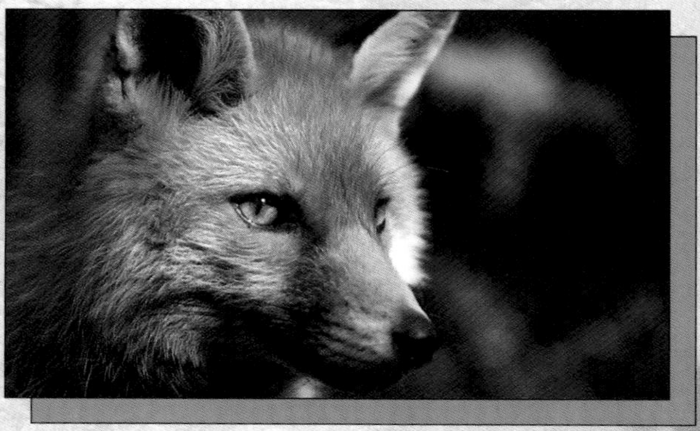

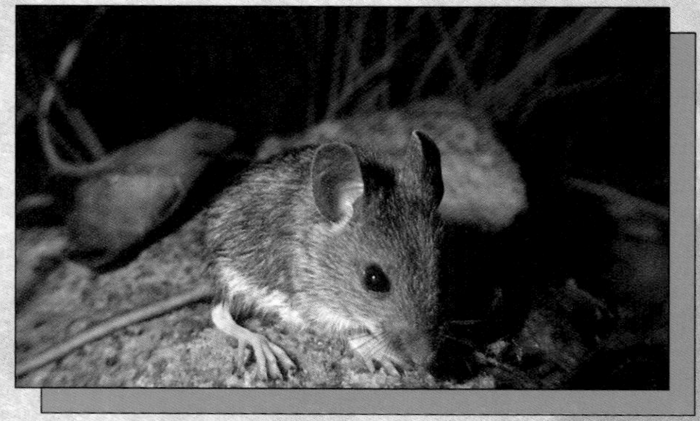

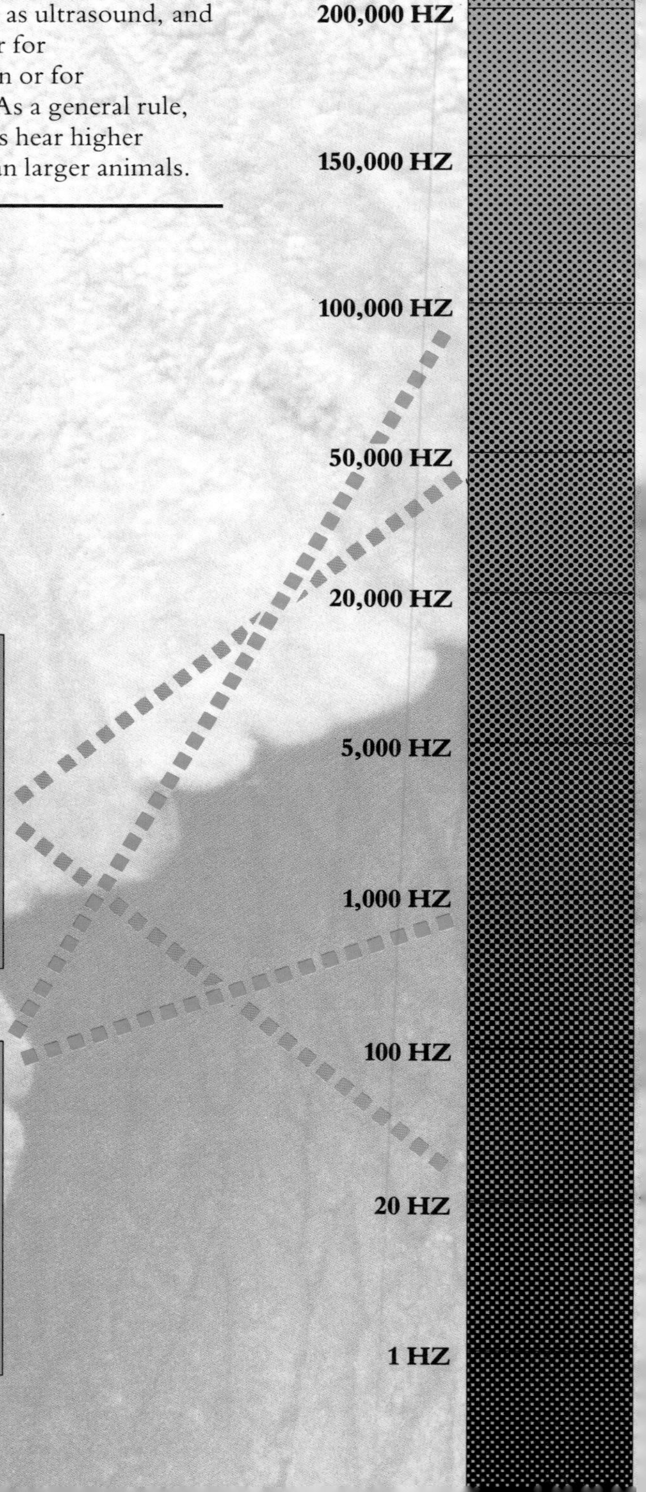

200,000 HZ

150,000 HZ

100,000 HZ

50,000 HZ

20,000 HZ

5,000 HZ

1,000 HZ

100 HZ

20 HZ

1 HZ

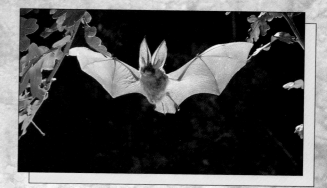

200,000 HZ

150,000 HZ

100,000 HZ

50,000 HZ

20,000 HZ

5,000 HZ

1,000 HZ

100 HZ

20 HZ

1 HZ

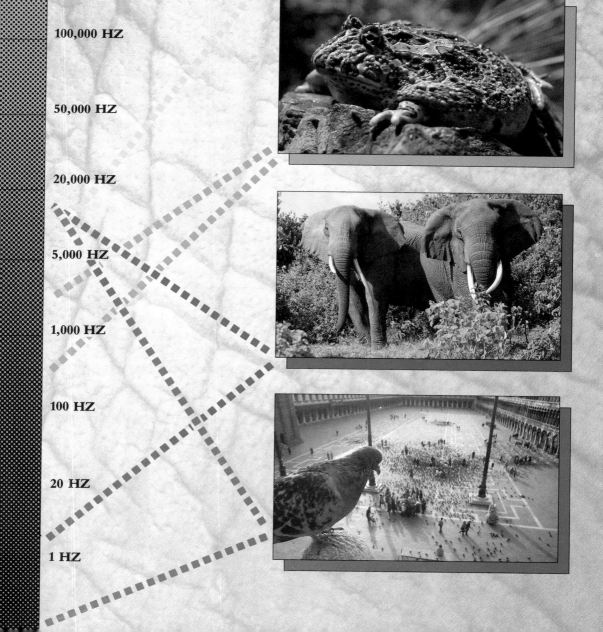

a different serenade. A male settles close to a female and identifies himself by vibrating his wings to the rhythm of his love song. If the female is of a different species, she emits a buzz and the male flies off to try his luck elsewhere.

The sound of its wings can be an insect's downfall, however, for some predators can also tune into it. The bolas spider lures moths with a scent, and catches them on a blob of glue at the end of a thread. The caira spider attracts insects in a similar way and then grabs them out of the air. Both spiders hunt at night, and the sounds of the insects' wingbeats are their only guide to the position of their prey.

Like those of some insects, a spider's ears detect the movement of air caused by a sound rather than the pressure waves. The ears are specialised hairs arranged in rows on each of the spider's eight legs. The frequencies that a spider's ear responds to depend on the length of the hairs. Large spiders have long hairs, which are tuned to the wingbeats of large insects, while small spiders have short hairs. The spider can judge the size of an insect by the loudness and frequency of its vibrations, and hides or runs away if the insect is too big to overpower. However, any sound within the correct range will attract it, even a person humming. Some house spiders have gained a reputation as music lovers by appearing whenever a particular tune is played on the piano. In reality, they are simply attracted by notes which evoke the sound of wings.

Although spiders and insects hear the world in a very different way from us, they are sampling the same sounds carried through the air. Huge numbers of creatures listen in to vibrations carried by another medium – water.

THE SOUNDS OF THE OCEAN

When the US navy used underwater listening devices called hydrophones to detect German U-boats during World War II, they were amazed to pick up barking, clicking and groaning noises. These were not the sounds of a new enemy vessel, but the calls of fishes. Until this time, many people imagined that the underwater world was silent. However, a sound source in the ocean can make water molecules vibrate in the same way as a noise on land causes the vibration of air molecules. In fact, sound travels much better in water than in air, as any diver will know. Divers may hear a motorboat apparently bearing down on them and then surface to find that the boat is actually a considerable distance away. Sea animals take full advantage of the efficient passage of sound through water, and the ocean is as full of sound as a woodland in spring.

Like birds, fish produce a variety of calls to attract a mate. The male bicolour damselfish flexes the muscles attached to its swim bladder as it patrols its patch of coral reef. This creates a chirping noise, and if a female draws near, he increases his rate of chirping to encourage her. A minnow, called the satinfin shiner, purrs, the cod grunts, while the haddock's love song resembles a motorbike and it will keep up its unmelodious call for 20 minutes at a time.

The sounds used to chase away competitors are equally diverse. If a male approaches, the damselfish's chirping changes to an aggressive popping noise. The grouper slaps closed the covers of its gills to create a booming sound. Other fish thump, drum or even growl to warn off intruders.

Some fish may use sound to communicate with their young, and to signal danger. But, as on land, any sound can also elicit danger. Trumpet fish may even locate their prey by listening out for fish's calls. Remaining silent may allow fish to evade these predators, but it is no defence against sharks and barracudas. These animals can detect the sound of a fish swimming, even hearing the sound of its muscles as they contract.

The underwater world vibrates with the noises of other creatures besides fish, including the snapping of shrimps and the clicks of barnacles. These high-pitched sounds are unlikely to be heard by passing fish, however, because although a few species, such as minnows, can hear as high as 8000 hertz, the majority are most sensitive to low frequencies and hear little above 500 hertz.

The ears of fish vary, but most are relatively simple. They follow different designs from our own, all of which allow them to tune in to water-borne sounds. Some ears detect the movement of water molecules created by a noise, while others sense its pressure waves. Often the swim bladder is involved in receiving sound and will act as an acoustic amplifier to sounds of the right resonant frequencies. The ear is connected to this air-filled chamber either through a special channel or a chain of small bones. Ocean mammals, such as seals and whales, used to live on land and had ears very similar to ours. Since they returned to the oceans, their ears have undergone changes to suit the needs of their marine home. Seals can close their earholes when they are underwater, and the earholes of whales have shrunk to a minute size. Although we need earholes to let in air-borne sounds, water-borne vibrations pass easily through the tissues of these sea mammals' heads to reach their ears.

Whales have excellent powers of hearing and, not surprisingly, a very elaborate repertoire of calls.

THE SONGS OF WHALES

The toothed whales, such as dolphins, sperm and killer whales, are expert hunters, preying on fish, squid and other large animals. They emit a variety of noises, many of them too high for us to hear. Within our range, there are pulses of sound resembling barks, squawks and groans, and the more social species also produce whistles from 0.5 to 2 seconds long.

The calls of killer whales vary from group to group and these dialects are so distinct

Both humpback whales (*right*) and dolphins (*bottom*) are known to produce a wide range of calls to communicate with other members of their species. In addition, dolphins produce high-pitched bursts of ultrasound (*see page 92*), building up a sort of X-ray sound 'image' of their prey (*below*) and the surrounding area from the complex reflections of sound they receive.

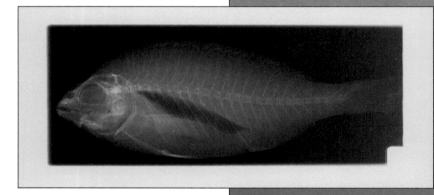

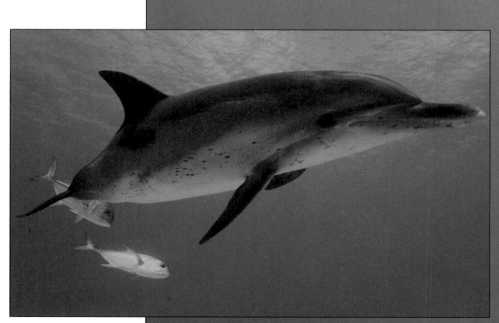

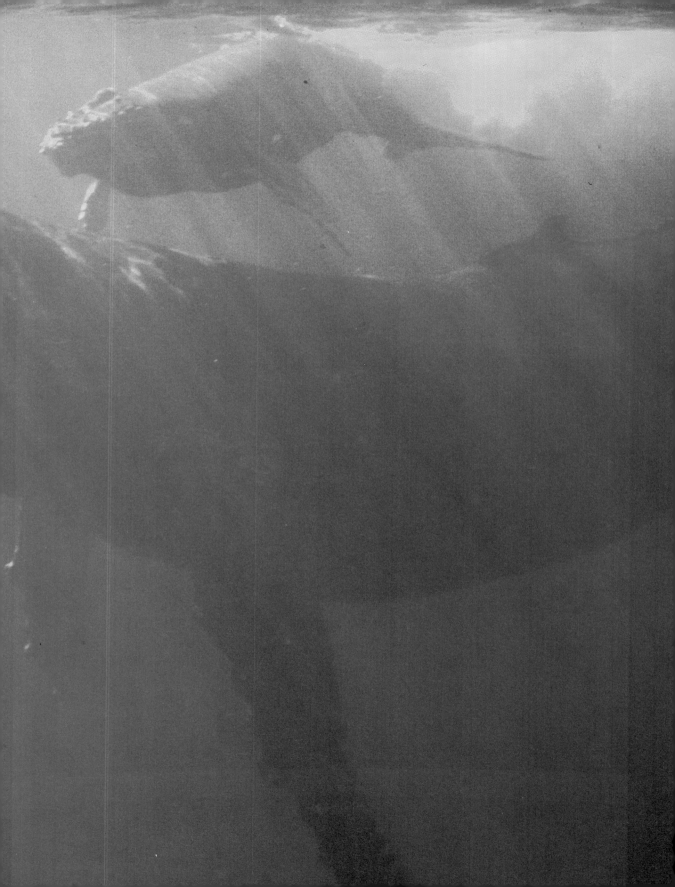

that people can tell them apart. The sperm whales and narwhals use a more sophisticated system in which each individual has a unique sound. These whales can presumably identify each other from their calls, and may even be exchanging much more information. Studies of dolphins have indicated that their communication is very complex, possibly as complex as human speech, but these sounds have proved difficult to decipher.

The other main group of whales, the baleen whales, browse around the surface of the ocean, filtering plankton through the vast, brush-like plates in their mouths. Their calls are also very intricate, and the sounds of some of them, the young, sexually mature humpback males, are so haunting that they have become a best-selling record.

The humpback's singing occurs mainly during the winter breeding season when hundreds of whales congregate. The songs contain up to eight themes, each one consisting of repeated phrases. A singing session may continue for 22 hours, incorporating many songs lasting from 8 to 20 minutes each. Again, the songs vary from group to group, but they also evolve over time. At the beginning of the season, portions of last year's song can still be heard. As the season progresses, additions, deletions and modifications create more complex compositions, with each member of the group singing a similar song. The humpback's singing can be heard from 32 kilometres away and so probably helps to bring breeding individuals together. What other significance these songs have remains a mystery.

After the breeding season, baleen whales disperse and individuals may be separated by hundreds of kilometres. At least one species, the fin whale, manages to communicate across these vast distances. Although its calls are very loud, we cannot hear them for they are at around 20 hertz, the lower limit of the human ear. This is the best frequency to use under pack ice, where fin whales spend some of their time; it also penetrates well through the open ocean. Exactly how far the fin whale's call travels is not known. It can probably be heard hundreds of kilometres away and could reach individuals thousands of kilometres away if the fin whale makes use of a channel in the ocean.

This channel occurs because the velocity of sound in sea water depends on the temperature, pressure and salinity of the water. As these change with depth, at about 1500 metres, these factors combine to form a channel of water which acts like a voice tube. Sound waves bounce off the sides of the channel as though they had hit solid walls, focusing the sound along the channel. In this way, sound can travel thousands of kilometres without weakening or dispersing.

The navy uses this channel for a system called Sofar (*sound fixing and ranging*) to, for example, track submarines. Fin whales are not known to descend to depths as great as 1500 metres. However, it is likely that they too could use the channel by bouncing their calls off the continental shelves which slope down into it. If so, their sounds now have to compete with the sounds of submarines in the Sofar channel. Nearer the surface, their communications may also have been seriously affected during this century by the low-frequency din of modern shipping.

CALLING LONG DISTANCE

The fin whale uses a low-pitched call because low-frequency sounds travel further than high-frequency ones. To understand why, imagine a sound source as a stick being dipped in water. At each dip, a wave spreads out from the stick across the water. If the rate of dipping is increased, the waves move closer together, while if it is decreased, the waves move further apart.

Sound waves are very different to water waves but the length of a sound wave changes with its frequency in the same way. Sound travels at about 340 metres per second in air. At a frequency of 20 hertz, there are 20 waves each second and so the length of each one is about 17 metres. Such long waves can pass easily around most objects. However, at the upper limit of our hearing, 20 000 hertz, the waves are only 17 millimetres long. These short waves cannot travel far because they bounce off even small objects. A common example of this is the annoying dull throb of a neighbour's stereo. The walls and windows absorb the higher-pitched melodies, while the monotonous bass and drums penetrate relentlessly.

Other animals exploit the carrying power of low frequencies, listening in to sounds below our range of hearing, called infrasound.

THE REALM OF INFRASOUND

Birds respond to a wide range of sounds but for many years it was assumed that their low-frequency hearing was poorer than ours. Then, using sensitive equipment in a laboratory, scientists found that pigeons can detect sounds as low as 0.1 hertz – that is, one vibration every ten seconds. Since pigeons' ears are not exceptional, it is likely that many birds can pick up infrasound. This discovery has led to much speculation about how birds use this phenomenal ability. The most intriguing possibility is that infrasound may be used by migrating birds as an aid to navigation.

Like many animals, birds build up a mental map of their home area from sight, sound and other cues. With infrasound, their auditory maps could extend for hundreds of kilometres around their home. Even far from home, they could gain clues to the positions of, say, sea, desert or mountain ranges from the differing sound patterns these features produce. Infrasound may also allow them to predict the weather.

During the dry season, male African guinea fowl live together in groups. Then, just before the rains come, they split up and establish territories for breeding. The rains do not come at the same time each year and yet the guinea fowl always seem to know when the wet season is about to begin. Their accurate predictions may be based on

◼ INFRASOUND AND BIRD NAVIGATION

◼ Extremely low-frequency sounds (infrasound) carry for hundreds of miles and birds that can detect these sounds may use them as a guide to navigation. Regular sources of infrasound, audible long before they become visible, may act as 'acoustic landmarks' which birds learn to recognise and use to pinpoint their direction.

◼ The infrasound produced by breaking waves *(above)* and the sands of some deserts, which 'hum' at an infrasonic frequency of 1 hz *(below)*, may be an important guide for any long-distance migrant as many birds cross vast expanses of sea and desert to reach their wintering grounds.

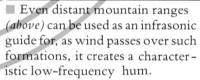

■ Even distant mountain ranges *(above)* can be used as an infrasonic guide for, as wind passes over such formations, it creates a characteristic low-frequency hum.

Man-made machinery makes towns and cities *(below)* a major source of low-frequency sound, while waterfalls *(bottom)* also produce infrasound. Birds may become familiar with such local sources and home in on them to find their way home.

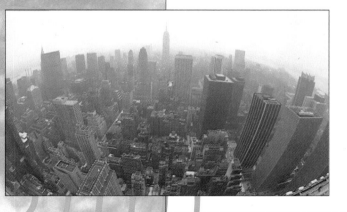

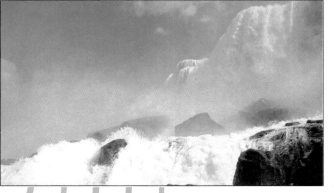

infrasound. We hear thunder when it is close enough for its highest frequencies to reach us, but it also generates infrasonic sounds which travel much further. By listening in to these, guinea fowl could hear storms hundreds of kilometres away and so have advance warning of a change in the weather.

The ability to predict, and so avoid, bad weather would be invaluable to migrating birds. However, any infrasonic vibrations they pick up on migration would be mingled with the very similar air movements produced by turbulence in the atmosphere, and some birds appear to take advantage of these as well. Known as pseudosounds, such movements occur, for example, in columns of air called thermals. As the sun heats the ground, pockets of warm air form which periodically break away and rise upwards in a column. Large migrating birds, such as storks, pelicans and cranes, rise up on these natural elevators and then glide off, losing height until they find another thermal. This is an extremely efficient method of long-distance travel, but just how these birds locate the thermals has always been a mystery. It now seems possible that they are guided by the low-frequency pseudosounds in the thermals.

Overlaying all these sounds are the wingbeats of the birds themselves. A bird the size of a sparrow beats its wings 14 times a second, while the larger gull beats its wings 3 times a second, so these are also at infrasonic frequencies. Tuning in to the wingbeats may help birds maintain their position in the flock, particularly at night.

Not only are some birds known to detect infrasound, but one species has been shown to produce infrasonic calls. Capercaillies are large black grouse which live in the coniferous forests of northern Europe. For most of the year they live solitary lives, scattered throughout the forest. However, during the breeding season, males gather together on a display ground known as a lek. There, as they strut with tails fanned, wings drooping and bills upstretched, they emit a strange mixture of clicking and gobbling noises. These calls sound very quiet to us and yet they attract females through kilometres of dense forest. When the noises were recorded, it was found that much of the call was at frequencies too low for us to hear, and it seems likely that the females were responding to this infrasound.

To find another animal with this ability we have to look outside the avian world to the largest land animal – the elephant. It has been known for a long time that, partly due to their immense size, elephants can hear much lower sounds than we can. However, no one was aware that they are also infrasound producers until recently, when a researcher at Washington Park Zoo felt a strange rumbling sensation coming from one of the elephants. Acting on a hunch, she brought in a low-frequency recorder and found that infrasound was emanating from its forehead. The sound was created in the larynx and propagated through air resonating in a hollow beneath this natural sounding board of the forehead. The animal tested was an Asian elephant, but it was soon confirmed that African elephants produce infrasound as well. The sounds were just below the limit of human hearing.

This discovery explained observations that had puzzled elephant watchers. A herd of elephants is often widely scattered across open bush or woodland. Yet members of the group immediately come to the help of an individual in trouble and, if danger threatens, the whole herd may simultaneously move away, apparently silently. By communicating through infrasonic calls, elephants can co-ordinate the movements of individuals several kilometres apart.

Both males and females use infrasound to attract mates, and when recordings of these calls were played, elephants were drawn towards the loudspeakers. A baby separated from its mother also uses infrasound, and when suckling it emits infrasonic versions of a human baby's gurgles.

At the moment we know little about the realm of infrasound and how animals exploit it. At the other end of the scale, however, our machines have picked up a host of animal noises at frequencies above the range of our ears, called ultrasound.

PRIVATE CHATTER

The familiar squeaks which we associate with mice and rats are the lowest sounds these rodents make. Their calls range from below the upper limit of our hearing, 20 000 hertz, into ultrasonic frequencies, some reaching as high as 100 000 hertz. Even if our ears could respond to sounds of this pitch, we would need to be very close by to eavesdrop on their conversations. Such high frequencies cannot travel far because they are rapidly absorbed by floorboards, undergrowth, or even by the air itself, particularly if it is foggy or misty. This makes ultrasound ideal for rodents, allowing them to chat privately in their enclosed runs and burrows without being heard by predators.

Most at risk are youngsters, which may even be attacked by adults of their own species. When touched by an adult mouse, a young mouse emits a special ultrasonic call that seems to have a soothing effect on the adult. The greatest danger for the very young is to be separated from the nest because they are helpless and can quickly die of cold. Isolated young mice squeak repeatedly at frequencies of 45 000 hertz to 88 000 hertz, until their mother comes and returns them to the nest.

Mice also produce ultrasound during mating, when the pelvic thrusts of the male are accompanied by rhythmic squeaks. The male rat croons a post-coital song consisting of bursts of sound between one and three seconds long that are only just above human hearing. When fighting, however, rats produce much higher sounds. If two strange males meet, they box and wrestle, emitting a succession of sounds at between 40 000 and 70 000 hertz, each lasting less than seven-hundredths of a second. Eventually, one rat adopts a submissive posture and its squeaks lengthen to about a second each, while

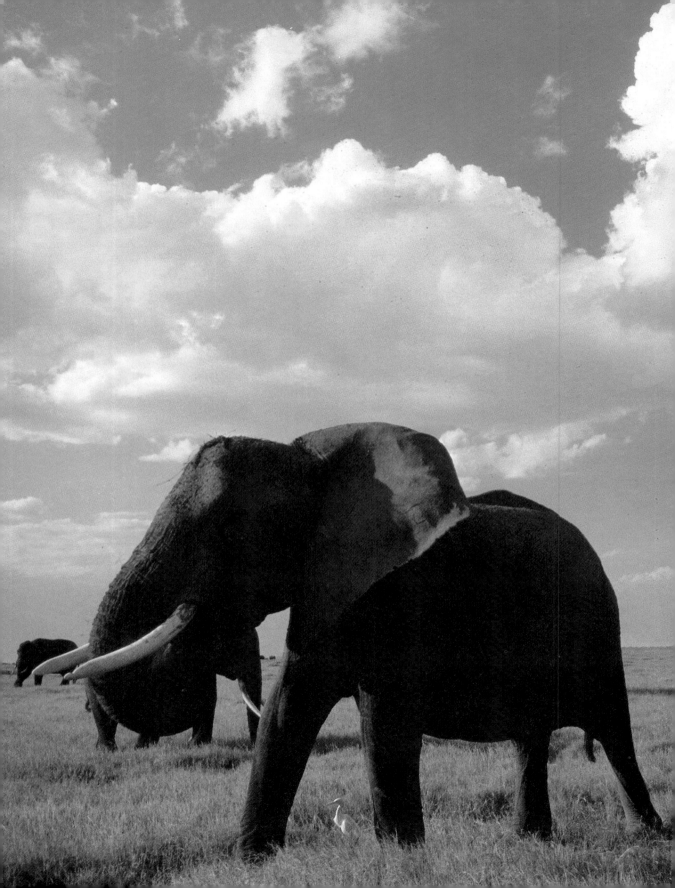

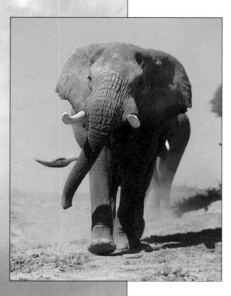

Elephants can hear much lower sounds than we can. It has recently been discovered that they also produce low-frequency sounds (infrasound), and it seems that they can use this to communicate with other members of the herd over vast distances.

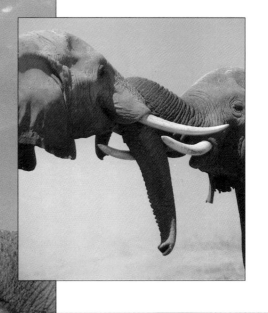

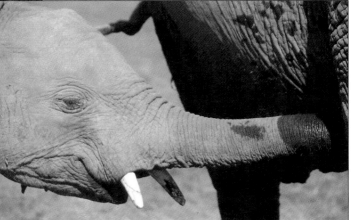

their pitch drops to about 30 000 hertz. This means that a dominant rat can be identified by its call, and so a rat colony can maintain its hierarchy without unnecessary fighting.

Some of these rats' calls may be heard by dogs, which can detect frequencies up to 40 000 hertz, while that expert mouser, the cat, can hear sounds as high as 70 000 hertz. Another popular pet, the hamster, can detect vibrations up to 100 000 hertz. Such high-frequency hearing offers an advantage in addition to privacy. The higher the pitch of a sound, the easier it is to locate. We can sense this even among the narrow range of sounds that we can hear. The low rumble of a juggernaut seems to vibrate all around us but we can immediately turn towards a high-pitched sound, such as a whistle being blown. The ability to accurately locate a noise is particularly important for the animals which use sound to find their way around.

GUIDED BY SOUND

Some blind people can walk unaided down a busy street without bumping into anything. One blind six-year-old could even steer a tricycle almost as skilfully as a sighted child. Such people describe their ability as being due to 'shadows' or 'pressure' felt on the face, and so the skill has come to be known as facial vision. However, when researchers plugged the ears of volunteers, their facial vision disappeared showing that they were actually being guided by sound. In fact, blind people sense objects by detecting the sounds reflected off them, particularly the sounds of footsteps.

Many sighted people also have experience in using sound reflections to judge distances. For example, by shouting into a pitch black cavern we can gauge its size from the time it takes the echo of the shout to reach us. Animals which spend much of their time in the dark use a more sophisticated system than us.

The cave swiftlet of south-east Asia roosts and breeds in caves, making a nest of saliva which is the main ingredient of birds'-nest soup. The oilbird of South America also spends much of its life in caves, and both birds fill their homes with the clicking of their calls. Even in total darkness, the birds can sense the walls of their cave and any other obstacles in their path by listening to the echoes of their clicks. Because the birds dart around quickly, they have to emit clicks and receive their echoes at a very fast rate in order to avoid collisions. The oilbird's click lasts for about a hundredth of a second and is not a single sound but a burst of pulses, each only about a thousandth of a second long. We hear the call as a click because our ear cannot discern the short pulses. The oilbird not only hears each pulse as a distinct sound, but can also interpret its echo.

The birds' echolocation is, however, limited by the frequencies that they can hear. The oilbird's hearing falls off rapidly above about 6000 hertz and it is most sensitive to sounds around 2000 hertz, which is the main frequency of its clicks. Unfortunately, sound waves at this frequency are quite long, and so instead of bouncing off small objects, they simply pass around them. Because of this, oilbirds cannot sense objects much smaller than 20 centimetres across. The cave swiftlet is more sensitive and can avoid objects as small as 6 millimetres.

Other animals, such as the Rousettus fruit bats, produce sounds at a higher frequency, although still within our range of hearing. By clicking its tongue, a Rousettus bat can locate objects only 0.5 millimetres across while flying at high speed. To achieve finer detail, animals would have to move up into ultrasonic frequencies, and a number of mammals have done just that.

Shrews and tenrecs emit echolocating calls as they go along their runs. Their ultrasonic squeaks or tongue clicks reflect off objects as small as grass stems and, supplemented by their other senses, help these animals find their way around. Their bursts of sound are very crude in comparison with the well-regulated clicks of the oilbirds and cave swiftlets, but are adequate to guide these much slower, ground-based animals. A group of aerial hunters has combined the use of ultrasonic frequencies with refined bursts of sound to produce extremely high resolution.

ULTRASONIC ECHOLOCATION

The insectivorous bats use such an intricate system of echolocation that they can pluck flying insects out of the air in total darkness. The sounds they produce in their larynx may reach as far up the ultrasonic scale as 200 000 hertz, allowing them to detect objects as tiny as a midge 20 metres away. Their huge pinnae, which can be swivelled round to scan the air, gather the echoes of the sound into the earholes. The bat's ear is similar in design to ours, but with refinements which give it great sensitivity at ultrasonic frequencies. Much of its brain is devoted to receiving and interpreting these ultrasonic messages, for the bat relies on its hearing to 'see' the area around it. The sound it emits scans the scene in front of it, rather like a beam of light, and its brain uses the echoes received to form a 'sound picture' of the scene.

When the bat hunts, it emits a string of pulses at a rate of about ten a second. If it detects an object, it improves definition by increasing the pulse rate to 25–50 per second, and as it swoops for the kill, the rate reaches an incredible 200 per second.

Many bats improve their sound picture by using different frequencies. Each pulse sweeps through a range of frequencies like an ultrasonic siren, for example, starting at 80 000 hertz and ending at 40 000 hertz. The lower frequencies penetrate further, scanning a wider area, while the higher frequencies bounce off very small objects. Using a range of frequencies also has the advantage that the different wavelengths reflect off different parts of an object, revealing fine detail.

A few bats in this group catch fish rather than insects, and use this technique to sweep the water. Although their pulses cannot penetrate the surface of the water, they reveal

■ BAT ECHOLOCATION

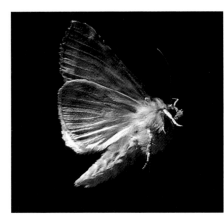

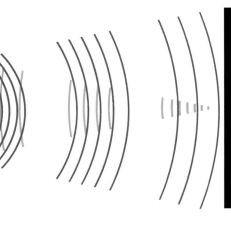

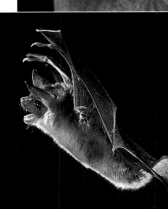

■ BASIC ECHOLOCATION

With this system, the bat produces sound in pulses and times the delay between emitting the sound and the echo bouncing back from the target. A long delay means the target is far away; a short delay means the bat is closing in. A flying bat normally creates between 5 and 20 pulses every second, but as it homes in on its prey the rate rises to 200 pulses each second.

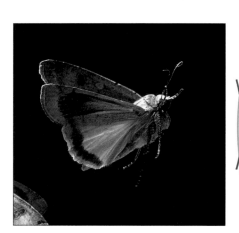

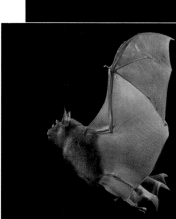

■ DOPPLER SHIFT

The bat creates a beam of ultrasound and then listens for the change in pitch of the echo. As the bat approaches the moth, it catches up on the reflected sound waves. The sound waves therefore appear to bunch together and, as the bat hears more sound waves each second, the pitch of the echo appears to rise. However, if the moth starts to fly away, the pitch of the echo begins to drop.

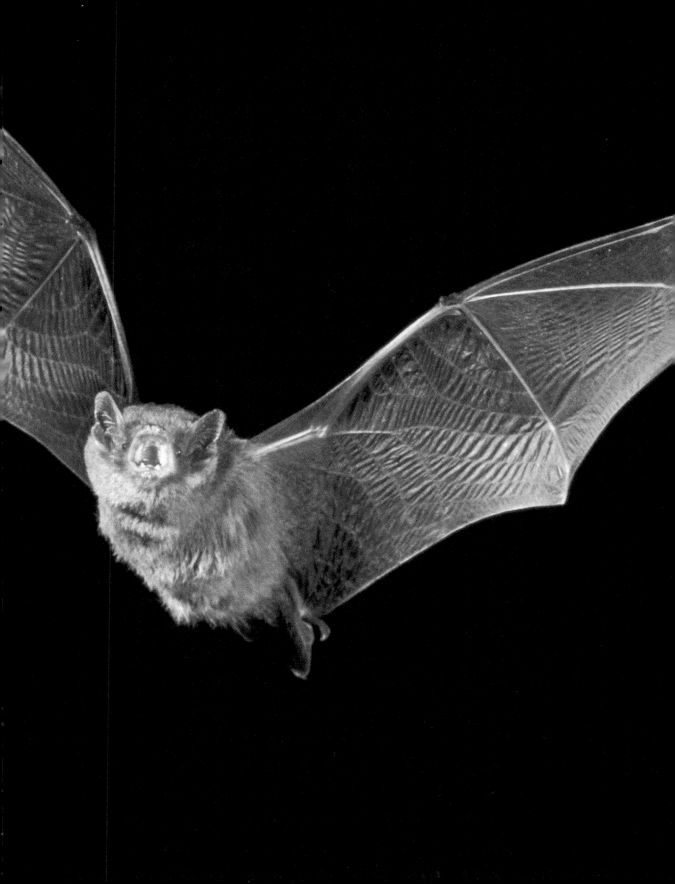

the tell-tale ripples of swimming fish. The bats can distinguish between the ripples created by, say, leaves and twigs, and those of prey, and swoop down to snatch fish out of the water with the large claws on their feet.

Some bats use a different method of echolocation, making use of what is known as the Doppler effect. This is the change in frequency of a sound that occurs when a source is moving relative to the listener. If a source is moving towards the listener the sound waves are bunched up and so seem higher, while if the source is moving away, the waves are spread out and seem lower. Anyone who has tuned into motor racing on the television will have heard this effect. As each car approaches the commentator's microphone the whine of its engine rises, and then starts to fall as the car passes the microphone and moves away round the circuit.

The bats which use the Doppler effect emit long bursts of sound. When chasing a flying insect, the bat can work out the direction and speed of the insect from the slight changes in frequency of the echoes bouncing off it. However, a bat may also use this technique in the same way as the police use radar. It conceals itself, and lies in wait for an unsuspecting moth. When a moth flies into range, it works out the exact speed and position of its victim and then flies out to pluck it from the air.

The insects are not entirely defenceless against this barrage of ultrasound, for many can hear the bats' sonic beams and take evasive action. The praying mantis has a single ear in the middle of its thorax which it uses for bat detection. The lacewing's ears are at the base of each forewing, and cause the wings to fold whenever they pick up the bats' echolocating sounds. Male lesser waxmoths and bush katydids call to their mates using ultrasound, but avoid being overheard by ceasing their courtship sounds as soon as they sense the approach of a bat. Noctuid moths and tiger moths respond by closing their wings and plummeting from the sky, or somersaulting out of the way. Tiger moths can also take their defence strategy a stage further, screaming out in ultrasound, which may jam the bats' sonar or warn of their foul taste.

The insectivorous bats are not unique, for another group of animals uses a very similar system – the toothed whales. These mammals often need to hunt in deep or murky water, where little light penetrates. The water in which river dolphins live is so muddy that they cannot see anything. As result their eyes have almost disappeared, but guided by sound alone they effortlessly catch their food.

The dolphins create their sounds in the larynx or in the passages leading to their blowhole. The sounds emanate from a dome-shaped structure on the head, known as the melon. This acts as a lens, but one that focuses sound instead of light. The returning echoes are believed to be picked up through the fatty interior of the lower jaw.

Like bats, dolphins emit pulses at a rate of 10–20 per second, increasing the rate to up to 200 per second as they home in on prey. They also produce similar frequencies, ranging up to 200 000 hertz. However, instead of sweeping through the frequencies with each pulse, the dolphins emit instantaneous bursts of sound containing a wide range of frequencies. From the complex reflections it receives, the dolphin can build up a detailed picture of the scene. It can also improve definition by tuning its frequency band to the object under investigation. The increased sophistication of the system used by dolphins is necessary because sound travels nearly five times as fast in water as in air. This means that at any frequency, sound waves in water are nearly five times as long as they would be in air, and so provide poorer resolution. The dolphin's echolocation system is good enough not only to allow it to find fish but also to select its favourite food.

Another effect of water-borne sound is that the dolphin 'sees' its prey very differently to the bat. The bat's air-borne clicks bounce off insects, whereas water-borne sounds pass through the tissues of a fish to the bone and swim bladder. So the sound image that a dolphin receives is more like an X-ray than a normal picture.

STUNNING WITH SOUND

Among the underwater chorus of singing fish and snapping shrimps are some animals equipped with a sonic weapon system. The pistol shrimp has a special claw which is held open at the hinge by two discs bound by suction. Closing the claw pulls the discs apart with a click that can be heard over a kilometre away. The effect of this on a nearby fish is devastating. The pistol shrimp then holds the disoriented fish in another claw, and fires a barrage of sound shots to its head before settling down to a quiet meal.

Sperm whales have been discovered which have such badly damaged jaws that they could not grab and hold a live fish, and yet these whales are otherwise healthy and well fed. One explanation is that they first immobilise their prey with sound. Such sounds could be generated by the spermaceti organ in the sperm whale's head. Muscles in this organ can produce massive air pressures, which could be concentrated into a sound beam with an intensity reaching 265 decibels. Fish and squid are killed in minutes by sounds much weaker than this. In comparison, our ears start to hurt at 150 decibels.

Certainly other toothed whales, the dolphins, can produce loud sounds. Among their repertoire of communication and echolocation pulses, dolphins in aquaria occasionally produce intense bursts of sound. When fired at a school of fish, these seem to act like a shotgun, disorienting many fish at the same time. Such a weapon would be particularly useful when dealing with a school, because the myriad moving bodies produce too confusing an echolocation picture for the dolphin to be able to single out a victim.

It is not yet known whether toothed whales regularly use such a weapon. If so, they combine a complex communication system and a detailed echolocation picture of their surroundings with the ability not only to locate and select prey but also to capture their meal with sound; the most versatile exploiters of sound in the natural world.

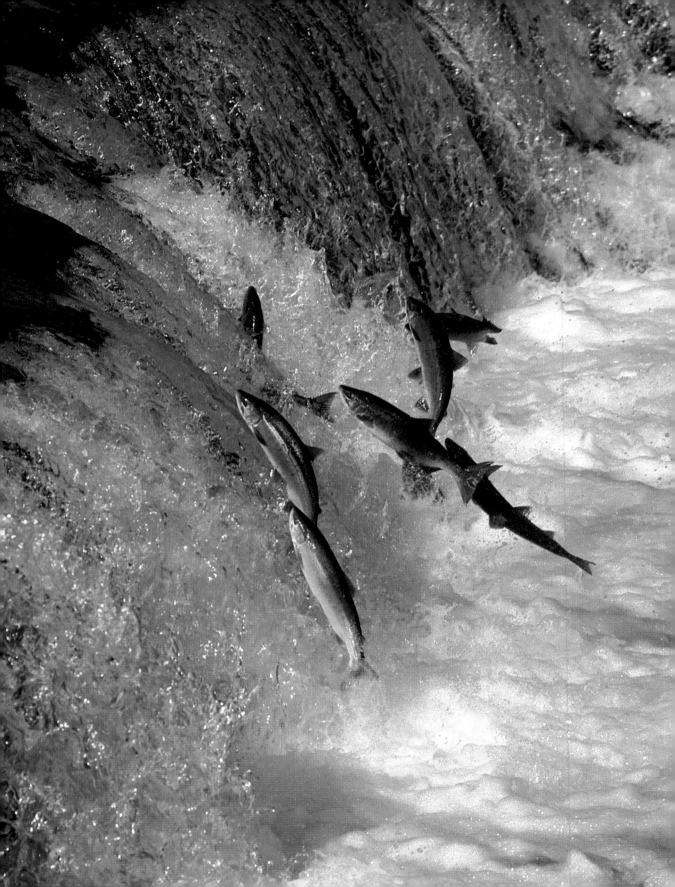

■ SUPER SCENTS

When our mouths water at the evocative aroma of good cooking, we are experiencing a sense found in even the most basic forms of life. Single-celled protozoa can detect the chemicals in their food and move towards them. Whether an animal is tasting or smelling its food may be difficult to determine, however, for the distinction between the two senses is often blurred. For example, the snake uses its forked tongue to gather scent particles from the air and tastes them on a special membrane, called Jacobson's organ, at the back of its mouth.

The smell and taste receptors of insects may be mingled, with some performing both functions. However, many have taste receptors on their mouthparts or feet, to identify the food they land on, while they find their food by detecting chemicals at a distance — the sense which we call smell. Usually, insects smell by tuning their antennae to scents in the air. The fragrance of flowers which we find so alluring acts as a magnet to bees. In return for its scent, the plant is rewarded with pollination, while the bee gains nectar. Other insects are attracted by scents which are much less obvious to us. Mosquitoes buzz around people's heads at night because they are drawn to the carbon dioxide which we give off as we breathe. Tsetse flies find the breath of cows equally enticing and can smell it from many kilometres away.

Fish have quite separate smell and taste organs but, unlike ours, their taste receptors are not confined to their mouths. The bodies of some catfish are covered with so many taste buds that they are almost swimming tongues, and they often use their taste buds to find their food. They can detect traces of distant chemicals in the water that passes through the nose, and some fish demonstrate amazing powers of smell. A trout can detect the smell chemicals of shrimp diluted a thousand million times, while the sensitivity of an eel is a thousand million times greater still.

Like mammals, birds have taste buds only on their tongues, and smell by sniffing the air. An oily mixture thrown from the back of a boat can draw hundreds of fulmars and petrels over kilometres of featureless ocean. Kiwis use their noses to find buried food, and recently it has been discovered that magpies and other birds do as well. The turkey vulture can detect a freshly killed carcass through kilometres of dense forest.

Similarly the polar bear can scent out a dead seal from 20 kilometres away. Most mammals use their sense of smell to find food, and all rely on smell to supplement their taste buds and bring out the full flavour of food, as anyone with a heavy cold will know. The sense of smell operates in the same way in all mammals, including us.

As we breathe, we draw air over an area of mucus-covered yellow tissue in the nose. In humans, this membrane contains about 10 million specialised cells, each bearing tiny hairs. Different sites on the hairs respond to particular scent chemicals, and the smell we experience depends on which combination of these sites is triggered.

Our membrane covers an area of about 4 square centimetres, which is small in comparison with many other mammals. Most cats have a smell membrane about 14 square centimetres in extent, while that of a dog may be as big as 150 square centimetres. Although our sense of smell does not compare as favourably as some of our other senses, it allows us to detect tiny traces of a very wide range of complex chemicals. It is surprising, therefore, that we are exceptionally limited in our use of smell. Many mammals rely on this sense more than any other, and scents have a profound effect throughout much of the natural world.

Smells are employed most widely to find food, but they also help many animals and plants to avoid being eaten.

THE SMELL OF DANGER

Grazing animals, such as deer and antelope, regularly break off from feeding and lift their heads to sniff the air for any scent of danger. Human hunters avoid detection by always approaching their prey from downwind. However, contrary to popular belief other predators, such as lions and cheetahs, never take wind direction into account when stalking, and the faintest whiff of them will cause a herd to become alert. This reaction to predators appears to be at least partly instinctive. The smell of lion's faeces makes red deer extremely nervous even though thousands of years have elapsed since the two species lived together.

Underwater animals are also tuned to the smells of their predators. Scallops and cockles usually lie motionless on the sea bed, filtering food out of the water. However, if a starfish approaches, queen scallops flap their shells and dance away, while spiny cockles extend their feet and flick themselves away. They react to a chemical present in starfish and will perform equally amazing gyrations if a piece of crushed starfish is dropped into the water. Similarly, an otter slinking into a stream 100 metres away from a trout will not go unnoticed. The skin of an otter, in common with that of all mammals, contains a substance known as L-serine, and fish are so acutely sensitive to this chemical that they can sense it diluted one thousand million times.

Unlike fish, the plant-like colonies of marine bryozoans cannot flee from danger. Instead, they grow a palisade of protective spines as soon as they scent a predator browsing nearby.

True plants are unable to perform this trick, but many can and do use scent to avoid danger. Some contain chemicals called pyrozines, the smell of which warns browsers that these plants taste unpleasant and should be avoided. This technique has been copied by insects, including ladybirds and certain moths and butterflies. Those which do not contain pyrozines naturally, gather them from noxious plants, either eating them as caterpillars or drinking them as adults. To advertise their unpalatability they don bright red and orange colours, which are recognised as warning signals by many predators.

Some moths take their defence a stage further by releasing a pyrozine froth from their abdomen to deter attackers. Skunks, polecats and martens use a similar strategy when threatened, producing a pungent, overpowering spray of more complex chemicals. However, the scents produced by danger usually have a very different purpose – to spread the alarm.

If someone gets stung close to a bee's nest, they are likely to find themselves quickly surrounded. The stinging bee will release an alarm scent, causing others to pour out of the hive and join in the attack. Far from the hive, though, the person will probably escape with only a single sting, because the same alarm chemicals cause the other bees to return to the hive.

Spraying the roses may also provoke alarm chemicals. That scourge of the garden, the greenfly, produces them when under attack, particularly from ladybirds. Although it dies, the greenfly's scent alerts its relatives to the danger, and they drop to the ground and escape. The wild potato exploits this behaviour in an ingenious defence. It frightens off greenfly by manufacturing their alarm chemicals itself. Unfortunately, we accidentally eliminated this system of protection when developing the King Edwards and other breeds of potato used today.

Most astonishingly, it has recently been discovered that many trees send out messages of danger when under attack from insects. On receiving these alarm chemicals, the sedentary neighbours increase the amount of tannin in their leaves, making them less palatable.

In contrast with these altruistic animals and plants, the behaviour of antelopes increases their own chances of survival. If a springbok or pronghorn antelope detects a hunting cheetah, it jumps up, releasing alarm chemicals from glands on its back into the air. An explosion of spectacular leaps and bounds ensues as the message spreads through the herd and the antelopes take flight. This not only provides a dazzling display which might confuse the predator, but also gives each antelope the advantage of safety in numbers within the fleeing herd.

When impala panic, they bound away making spectacular leaps from side to side, kicking their back legs into the air. These leaps can be over 3 metres high, and the accompanying kicks release scent from glands on their fetlocks into the air. These scents not only communicate the alarm to the rest of the herd but may also produce an aerial

Reindeer regularly stop and sniff the air to detect approaching predators such as wolves. As they flee they release a scent that spreads alarm to the rest of the herd.

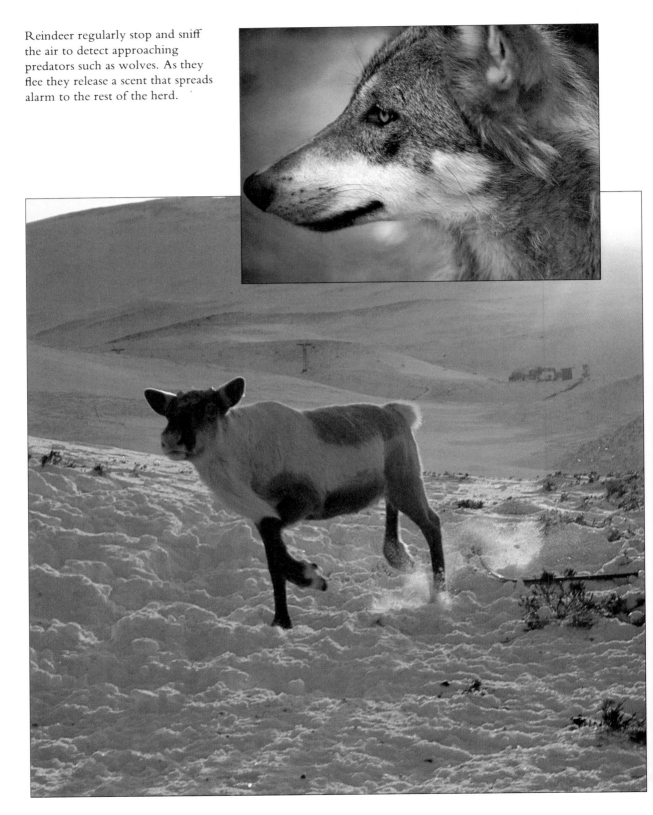

Similarly, when impala detect a hunting lion, they bound away, making spectacular leaps from side to side and kicking their back legs in the air. This releases scent from glands on their fetlocks into the air.

trail which other impala can follow without having to break their flight to sniff the ground.

Just as antelope release alarm scents from glands, all mammals secrete their scents through special glands of varying design, dotted around their bodies.

THE SMELL PRODUCERS

Our bodies are continually manufacturing chemicals to make us the smelly creatures nature intended us to be. The most powerful secretions are produced by our apocrine glands, which switch into action at puberty and turn off at menopause. These glands are concentrated in the hairier parts of our bodies and the hairs play a vital part in smell production. The apocrine secretions are diluted by sweat, and then acted upon by bacteria living in the protective jungle of hairs, to form distinctive body odours. The hairs also help to disperse the newly formed scents round the body.

We use a vast range of soaps and deodorants to attack our bodies, particularly those areas containing apocrine glands, in an often vain attempt to eliminate these odours. In this we are unique. Other mammals not only tolerate but revel in their smells, employing them in a wide variety of ways. They all have many different scent-producing glands on their bodies, the exact positions varying from animal to animal. In the majority, they are concentrated round the genital and anal regions, but hyraxes have them on their backs, deer on their legs, while pigs carry them on their knees. Many also have powerful glands on the head, those of cats being on their cheeks, those of elephants in front of their ears, and the horse even has one in its nose.

Some mammals' glands are more elaborate than our own and open into special pouches or pockets. This makes it easier for them to smear their secretions around, leaving scent messages for other animals. The brown hyena deposits two different smell chemicals by everting an anal pouch and squeezing it round grass stems. The anal pouch of that giant rodent, the capybara, contains a forest of easily detachable hairs, each covered with a hard crystalline secretion, which shower onto any object it touches.

An even more efficient method of dispersal is to add smell chemicals to the body's waste products. Hippopotamuses spread their scents by whisking their tails as they defecate, while white rhinos stamp in their faeces and then deposit the odour with each fragrant footstep.

However they are dispersed, all these scent messages convey information to other animals, particularly concerning territory.

TERRITORIAL MARKING

Many people try to discourage their pet tom cats from spraying but with little success. Tom cats spray the furniture as effectively as their relatives, male lions, spray the vegetation in their home. Lions then use their feet to paddle the urine into the grass. Rabbits register their presence with piles of droppings, as do badgers and spotted hyenas.

All of these animals have particular areas where they rest and breed, and some even feed within well-defined boundaries, seldom leaving their territory. Their scent markings help to familiarise them with their territory, and give them a sense of security. They also act as a badge of ownership, particularly to other males of the same species.

Animals which do not have a territory mark relatively seldom. Among territorial animals some, such as red foxes and mongooses, mark throughout their range, while coyotes and rabbits concentrate their scents along their territorial boundaries. As these animals roam around their home ground, any unaccustomed mark alerts them to the passage of a stranger. Similarly, an intruder immediately knows that the area is occupied, and can tell from the freshness of the scent how recently the owner has been there.

These smell messages allow animals to avoid unnecessary skirmishes. The intruder is able to recognise the owner because it smells the same as its mark, and so can decide whether to challenge for ownership or simply move on. To make this system more effective, animals emphasise their own scent by marking themselves as enthusiastically as their territories.

Hartebeests rub the glands by their eyes along the sides of their bodies, while deer rub their antlers on vegetation previously coated with their own scent. Chamois drench themselves in perfume by shaking their bodies as they urinate, and camels use their tails to whisk their urine into an odorous shower. A male rabbit goes even further and sprays the female with his urine as he leaps over her. Some animals, such as the bushbaby, exploit the scent of their urine for a very different purpose.

LAYING A TRAIL

Before a bushbaby sets out into the African night, it performs a strange ritual: it cups its hands and then urinates on them. In this way, it ensures that every step of its outward journey leaves a pungent reminder to guide it back home. Slow lorises use urine in a similar way and, in the laboratory, they will follow a trail smeared on the ground. Rats and mice leave trails along well-travelled routes by smearing secretions from glands on their body along the ground. Many antelopes have glands on their feet which leave odorous signposts wherever they go. However, the expert trail layers are undoubtedly the social insects.

Wherever army ants go, they leave a chemical trail for other ants in their group to follow, creating a huge foraging column radiating out from the nest. Most ants, though, only lay a trail when they have found a source of food. They deposit scent from the tip of their abdomen along the route from the food to the nest, and this trail is followed and added to by other ants as they return with food. The smell chemicals evaporate

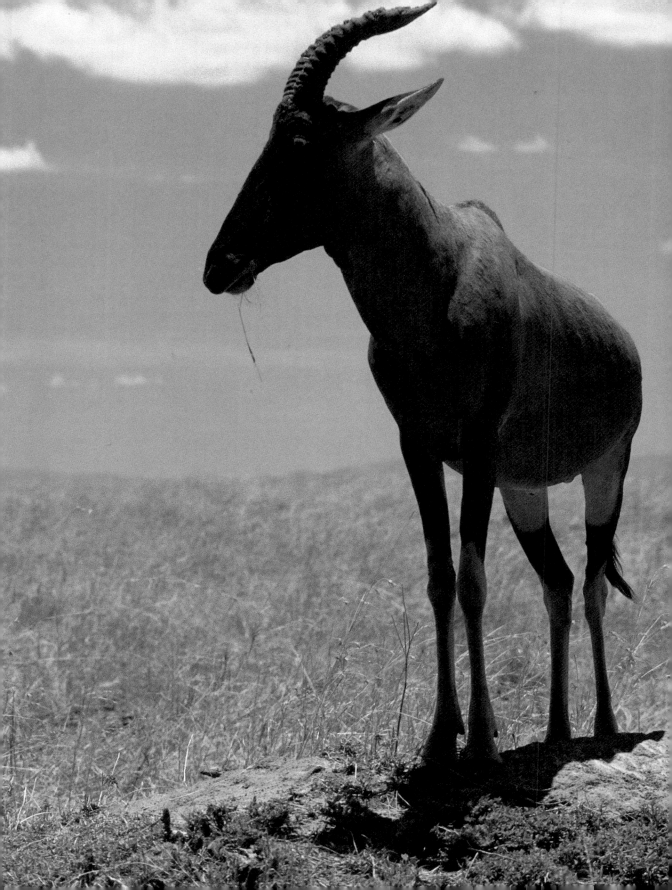

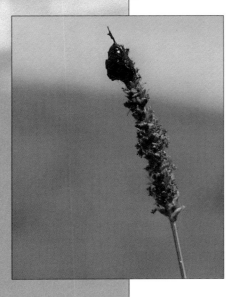

Antelopes are territorial animals and use scent markings to define their territory. Some of these scents are produced from a special gland just below the eye (*bottom*). When this gland is rubbed against a grass stem (*below*), it leaves a sticky deposit (*left*). An intruder matches this smell to the owner of the territory before deciding whether to challenge it to a fight.

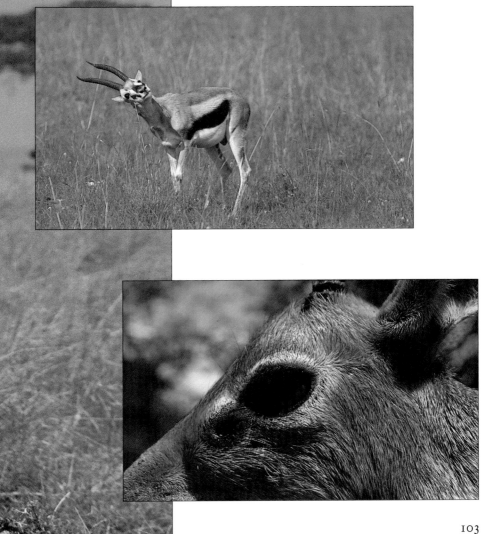

quickly and disappear without continual reinforcement, so the trail does not persist to mislead the ants once the food is exhausted. Ants such as leaf cutters, which use reliable supplies of food, lay more permanent scent trails and these may last for many months.

Some tropical bees send out scouts to find new sources of food. When they are successful, the scouts deposit scent on the tips of vegetation along the flight path to the nest, creating an aerial trail. They may also smear a marker scent on a flower which acts as a beacon to other bees.

More amazing still are the skills of those animals which can travel vast distances guided by scent, without even laying a trail.

THE SCENT OF HOME

Salmon lay their eggs in the gravel bed of fast-moving streams or rivers. The young parr which hatch out are dull-coloured, making them difficult to see in their freshwater home. However after one to three years a signal, possibly hormonal, causes them to don the silvery camouflage of sea fish. Each year, millions of parr undergo this dramatic transformation and head off downriver to the open ocean. After two to three years there, another signal prompts the now adult salmon to change hue again and return to fresh water to spawn.

The most remarkable feature of this migration is that each stream maintains a distinct population of salmon, sometimes visibly different from those in a neighbouring stream. This means that the fish not only navigate across hundreds of kilometres of ocean to the area of their birth but even locate the precise stream where they were spawned.

Although the fish are probably using water currents, the sun or a magnetic sense to help them achieve this feat, it has long been suspected that smell is also involved. The proportions of different chemicals of sea and fresh water vary slightly from area to area. Remembering these could supply the salmon with a smell map of its route across the ocean which might supplement its other senses. Certainly, salmon seem to use smell to guide them on the last stage of their journey. Detecting the scent of their natal stream in the waters flowing into the ocean causes the salmon to head inland, struggling up steep rivers or even rapids to reach the smells of home.

Exactly which smells salmon use to identify their natal stream is uncertain. Salmon can recognise their relatives by smell, showing that each population has a genetically distinct odour. Some researchers have suggested that mature salmon return simply by following the trail left by the young smolts swimming towards the sea. However, the journeys of smolts and mature salmon are often separated by several months, and so the smolts' odour would have to be very persistent to act as a guide. Other researchers think it is more likely that the fish remember the chemical composition of their home stream, and so pick up its scent in the open ocean.

Evidence for salmon's use of smell was provided by salmon reared in tanks containing minutes amounts of synthetic chemicals. Much later, these salmon were released into a lake and left to mature. When the fish were ready to spawn, the same chemicals were added to some of the streams feeding the lake. The salmon swam up only those streams which had been chemically scented.

As well as being important in the homing of fish, scent guides many amphibians to their ponds, and it may help turtles to find their nesting beaches. It is even possible that the most famous migrants of all – the birds – follow the scents of home.

Shearwaters and petrels are known to use smell to find their way back to their nests. However, these birds have particularly large nostrils, giving them an exceptionally good sense of smell for a bird, and their nests are often putrid. Until recently, it was assumed that other birds rely on different clues to guide them home. Then it was discovered that birds such as pigeons and swifts have difficulty navigating if their sense of smell is damaged. This find led to much speculation about what scents these birds might follow.

Some people think that, like shearwaters, pigeons and swifts fly towards the scent of home, although they would only be able to detect this over short distances. Others suggest that the birds are able to use their sense of smell over longer distances by remembering the scents of the prevailing winds. To test this, pigeons were kept in a loft, and olive oil was added to the wind blowing from the south, while turpentine was added to the wind blowing from the north. The pigeons were then split into two groups, one of which had their bills smeared with olive oil and the other with turpentine. On release, the pigeons showed that they had learned the smells associated with the different compass bearings. They assumed that they had been moved into the area these smells were coming from and, in an endeavour to return to the loft, those with olive oil on their bills flew north, while those with turpentine on flew south.

This test and many other experiments on the importance of smell in bird migration have been carried out in Italy. However, in other parts of the world, birds have responded differently to the same or similar tests. This may be because birds find scent cues particularly reliable cues in Italy, whereas in other parts of the world alternative guides are more important. The odours of the sea could be involved, and those birds living close to the coast might find smell particularly useful.

Whatever scent they follow birds, in common with many other animals, rely partly on their sense of smell to find their way. In contrast, we detect many odours as we travel around but seldom, if ever, use these as signposts. We are surrounded by animals which keep track of their fellows by scent yet we cannot even smell a human trail, let alone follow it. However, we have bred an animal that can.

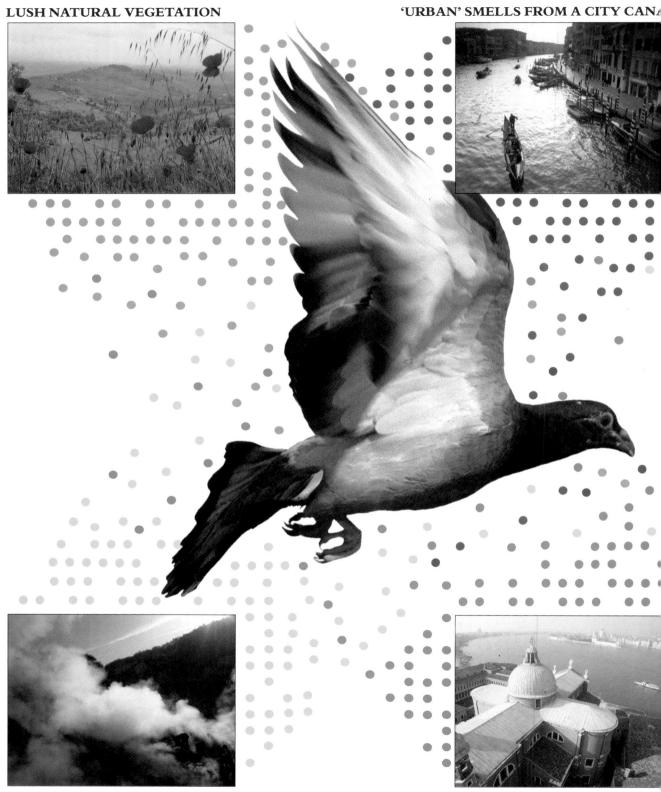

LUSH NATURAL VEGETATION

'URBAN' SMELLS FROM A CITY CAN

PUNGENT VOLCANIC ACTIVITY

THE GRAND CANAL – A COMBINATIO
OF SEA AND FRESH WAT

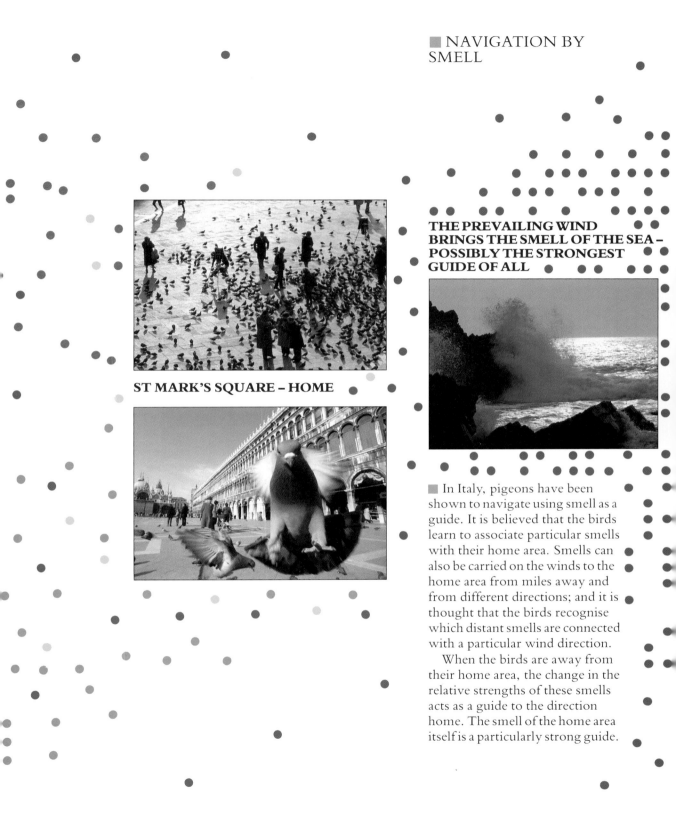

■ NAVIGATION BY SMELL

ST MARK'S SQUARE – HOME

THE PREVAILING WIND BRINGS THE SMELL OF THE SEA – POSSIBLY THE STRONGEST GUIDE OF ALL

■ In Italy, pigeons have been shown to navigate using smell as a guide. It is believed that the birds learn to associate particular smells with their home area. Smells can also be carried on the winds to the home area from miles away and from different directions; and it is thought that the birds recognise which distant smells are connected with a particular wind direction.

When the birds are away from their home area, the change in the relative strengths of these smells acts as a guide to the direction home. The smell of the home area itself is a particularly strong guide.

107

THE TRACKER DOG

Each day each of us sheds 50 million skin cells which rise on the warm air produced by the body and then fall to the ground forming a trail like a microscopic paper chase. We cannot sense these faint chemical traces, but the bloodhound can smell them immediately. Its secret lies in the fact that it has been selectively bred over centuries to reach the heights of scent detection.

Its long dewlap and floppy ears help to cup the scent as the bloodhound's nose passes over the ground. The long domed nose contains a smell-receptive membrane spread over rolled-up scrolls of bone. This membrane covers as much as 150 square centimetres in comparison with the 4 square centimetres in our own nose. In addition, the bloodhound has been bred to be particularly attuned to human smells. As a result, it is about a million times more sensitive to our trail than we are.

The bloodhound's nose may be so overwhelmed by the scent of fresh skin cells that it is unable to follow them. However, after about half an hour, some of the smell chemicals have started to evaporate creating an odour gradient, and the dog can set off on the trail. Other clues, such as the smell of crushed vegetation, help the tracker dog in its search.

The bloodhound can distinguish between the trails of different people. It follows unerringly the footsteps of a particular individual, even if a closely related person continually crosses their path. This is because the smell of each person – and, indeed, each mammal – is as unique as a human fingerprint.

SMELLS OF IDENTITY

Even the cleanest body is home to millions of bacteria which convert the glands' secretions into body odour. This bouquet is partly inherited, and so the bloodhound can occasionally be confused by the criss-crossing trails of identical twins. It is also affected by diet and people who regularly eat the same foods develop similar odours. However, there is still a slight difference between closely related people with similar habits, and among others the difference is so pronounced that even we can detect it.

In an experiment, people were given three identical T-shirts to smell and asked to select the one that they had worn. Three-quarters were able to distinguish between the T-shirts and pick out the one with their body scent on. When confronted with ten identical T-shirts, over half could still detect their own odours.

In similar experiments, mothers could select T-shirts worn by their children. Generally, women become familiar quickly with the scent of their infants, and can recognise their baby by smell alone only a few days after birth. However, a mother who is in contact with her baby immediately after delivery is much more likely to be able to do this than one who is not given her baby until a few hours after the birth. For many mammals, the smell bond built up during the few hours after birth is crucial.

A young wildebeest is able to run almost as soon as it is born, for it must be able to keep up with the other wildebeest when they flee a predator. In such a stampede, though, the baby sometimes gets separated from its mother. If this happens before the smell bond has been formed, the mother will not recognise the baby and will reject it when they meet again. The power of the smell bond is used by farmers to rear orphan or rejected lambs. The farmer can persuade a ewe which has lost her own lamb to accept another by tying her dead lamb's skin onto it.

The human baby's sense of smell develops gradually, and after about 10 days an infant can identify the smell of its mother's breasts. The numerous young of mammals such as rabbits and cats can even identify the particular nipple allocated to each and find it by smell within seconds of their mother returning.

The close relationship and constant contact between a mother and her baby make their smells very similar. In T-shirt tests, like those above, unrelated people could detect this similarity and match the odour of a baby to that of its mother. Such family odours are common in the animal world, and many animals extend them by deliberately merging their individual smells to produce an identifiable group odour.

When a cat rubs its cheek against its owner's leg, it is not just being friendly. The glands on its face are bestowing the cat's personal scent, making its owner smell pleasanter and more familiar. In the wild, lions regularly rub their heads against each other, transferring their individual scents to create an odour of the pride.

Kangaroo rats merge their smells by sharing a communal sand bath. Mongooses go further and rub their anal pouches on the same marking spot. This spreads smell-making bacteria from one individual to another. Combined with the fact that the members of a group have a very similar diet, all these activities produce a common smell of identity.

These group smells help to keep cohesion within the group and allow intruders to be detected easily. Their use is most developed in the social insects, where each nest has a unique odour. Any insect that arrives bearing the wrong smell is instantly attacked. Like many firm's security codes, the nest odour changes daily. Any worker away from the nest for more than a day will find that its smell identification badge has expired, and it will be killed.

Although group odours blur individual's scents, they cannot mask them entirely. In particular, males and females can usually be distinguished, and many emit such powerful sexual scents that they can be identified from kilometres away.

SEXUAL LURES

By sniffing the air, a dog can tell the sexual condition of any bitch in the neighbourhood and, if let loose, will follow the scent lure of a female on heat. Vixens attract foxes in

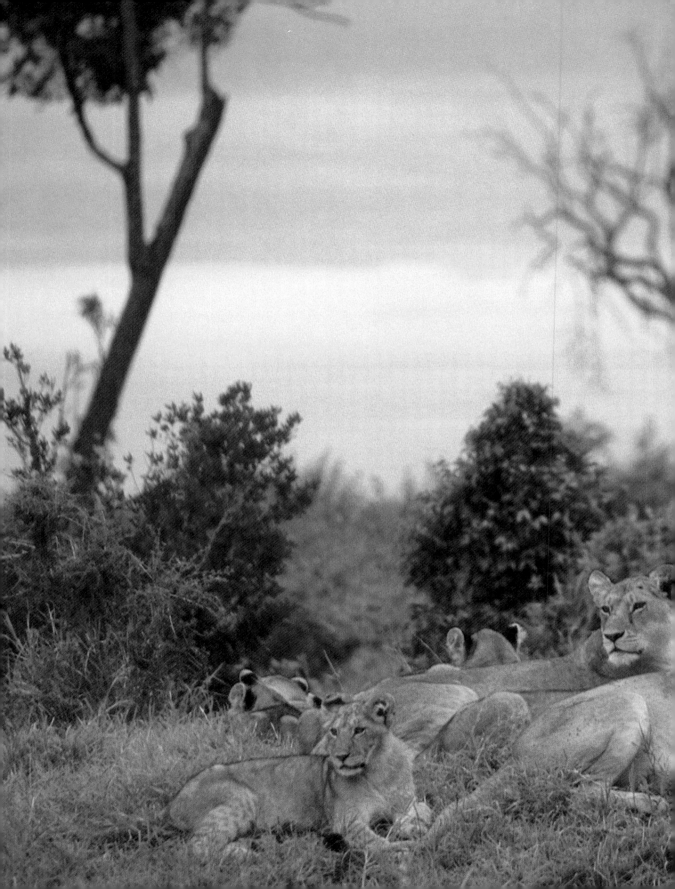

By rubbing their heads against each other, lions transfer their individual scents to other members of the pride. This creates bonds between members of the group and enables them to detect intruders easily.

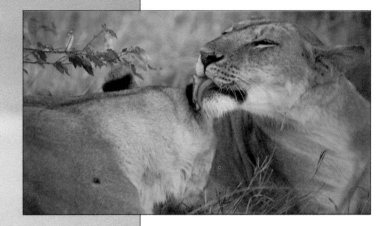

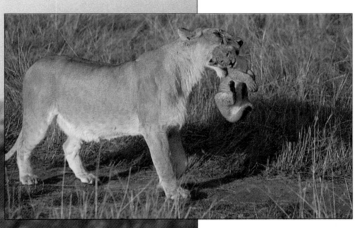

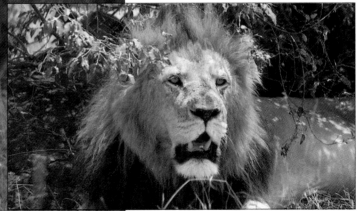

a similar way. Since the female is only on heat for a few days and the males are often widely scattered, these scents are vital for bringing the sexes together at the right time.

Some insects send out much longer-range messages. The female emperor moth puffs her sexual perfumes out from her abdomen, and these carry downwind in an expanding cone. Although the perfume is rapidly diluted by the air, the male's antennae are so sensitive that he can detect a female from as far as 5 kilometres away. The antennae are divided into large feathery plumes covered with tiny sensory hairs which are tuned to the female's smell molecules. Pores along the hairs filter out molecules of the right size and these are analysed. The detection of just one molecule of the female's scent causes the male to drop everything and fly upwind. If he loses the trail, he turns and flies across the wind until he picks up her scent again.

In some moths, the male emits the signal and the female responds, while both sexes of saltmarsh moth send out lures. This draws together large courtship parties, at which the females pick out the mates they prefer. Male cotton leafworm moths fare better, because the first to arrive at the female releases a scent which acts as a jamming signal on its competitors. The male oriental fruit moth employs greater subterfuge by producing a scent similar to the female's as soon as he arrives on the scene. This causes such a confusion of sexual identity for later moths that the first to arrive wins out.

Some reptiles use an even more devious strategy. Female garter snakes often lure so many suitors with their scents that the males form a frenzied writhing ball. A few of the males may then mimic the female's odour. These perfumed transvestites draw away rival males and sneak back to mate with the females. Not content with this, a successful male inserts a chemical plug in the female which prevents other males mating with her and causes any male which sniffs it to become impotent for days.

Other animals win their mates by producing powerful aphrodisiacs. As the male queen butterfly hovers in courtship, a delicate brush appears at the tip of his abdomen and sprinkles the female with perfumed scales. This dust has a magical effect on the female, who cannot resist its scent. Intriguingly, the aphrodisiac contains a chemical that the butterfly cannot manufacture and so, in order to create his perfume, the male must gather the vital ingredient from a particular withered flower.

Many moths also use aphrodisiacs, and have elaborate organs to release their exotic scents, such as hairs, brushes and large, inflatable sacs. The oriental fruit moth releases its perfume from white brush-like hairs on top of its abdomen and then fans the fragrance towards the female.

The two-lined salamander has a much less delicate approach. With its dracula-like teeth, it injects a potion directly into the female's bloodstream, and she immediately succumbs. The subtler newt waves its tail at the female and then trembles it provocatively, setting up ripples in the water which carry the aphrodisiac to her. If successful, he presents her with a package of sperm and she collects this in her vent.

Among mammals, the smell of the female's vagina is often the most powerful aphrodisiac. Hamsters will try to mate with anything smeared with this scent, while the gorilla always sniffs the female's vagina before attempting to mate. The vaginal scent also lets the male know whether the female is on heat, as does her urine. Red deer stags regularly sniff a hind's urine to detect the single day when she is in season. The male camel drinks the female's urine, swilling it in his mouth like a wine taster to assess her sexual state.

The most dramatic effects, though, are caused by scents which can actually alter the sexual state of individuals, particularly those living in close communities.

GROUP SEX

The nests of social insects are run almost entirely by smell, because in these dense communities it is the most efficient way of sending messages. When termites build their colony a scent is deposited in each globule of mud, guiding other termites to the spot. At the control centre there is usually a single queen, whose odours permeate the entire nest. Her scent messages stimulate the workers to groom and feed her, and prevent them from developing ovaries. If she dies or leaves, they are instantly aware of it, and soon develop eggs and start constructing cells ready for the new queen. The queen termite even releases a guide scent which determines the exact dimensions of the queen chamber. If soldier termites are killed in an attack, the decrease in the concentration of their scent causes the young females to develop into soldiers instead of workers.

In the parched and arid regions of East Africa dwell strange mammals which live in groups very like those of the social insects. Known as mole rats, these wrinkled, hairless rodents form subterranean communities of about fifty individuals. The smallest perform most of the work, such as digging and foraging for food. The medium-sized ones help with some of these tasks, while the largest spend all their time tending the young. The colony is ruled by a single queen, who again controls the sexual state of the community with her scent messages. These are passed through the toilet area which all the mole rats share.

Although less rigid in their organisation, other rodent communities are strongly affected by sexual odours. The scent of male lemmings communicates their social standing, and may change after a fight. The females can literally smell success, and will only mate with a victorious male.

Among mice, the merest whiff of a male can have a devastating effect. A female's reproductive hormones are triggered instantly and within 20 minutes her uterus starts to swell. If the female is pregnant, and the odour is that of a strange male, her embryos are either re-absorbed into her body or aborted. Immature females reach puberty 20

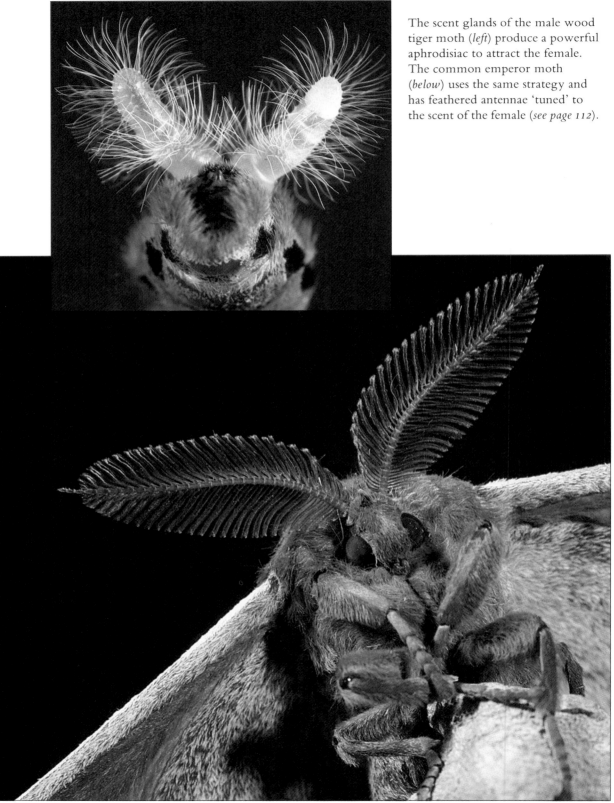

The scent glands of the male wood tiger moth (*left*) produce a powerful aphrodisiac to attract the female. The common emperor moth (*below*) uses the same strategy and has feathered antennae 'tuned' to the scent of the female (*see page 112*).

As termites build their mound, they lay down a scent to guide other workers. The special odour of the queen termite (*top right*) controls the whole colony. The balance between different types of termites is maintained by the distinctive smell of each 'caste': if large numbers of major soldiers, for example, are killed off, the decrease in this particular odour triggers the young in the nursery area (*bottom right*) to develop as major soldiers to replace the insects that have died.

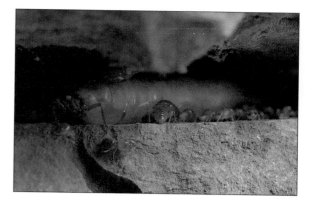

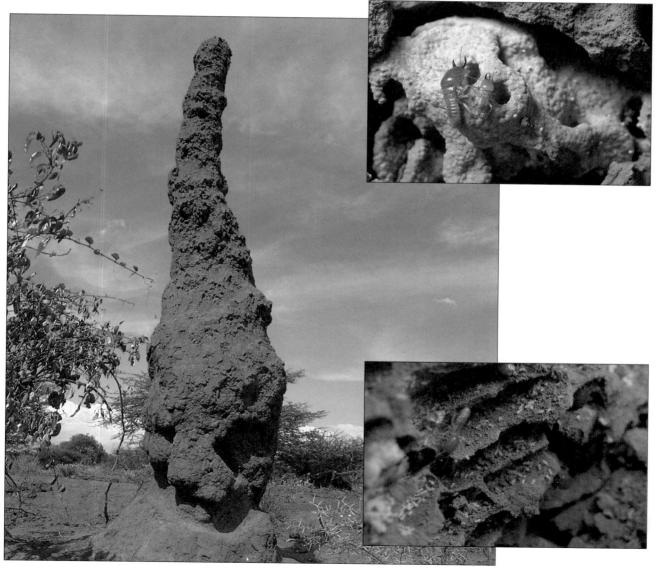

days earlier than when alone, and the puberty of young males is delayed. In this way, a dominant male can adjust the sexual state of the entire community to his benefit, through his scent alone.

This power is common among other mammals. The odour of the male affects the sexual cycles of female sheep, goats, coypus and some monkeys. Sexual scents even seem to influence the cycles of those mammals which try hardest to suppress their odours – us.

Women that live communally, for example in a college hall of residence, often find that their monthly periods become synchronised, and experiments have shown that the controlling force behind this is odour. In one study, the essence of secretions from a female's armpit were smeared onto the upper lips of other females who, perhaps fortunately, were not told of the origin of the smears. This continued each day for three months, by which time the cycles of the recipients had adjusted to the rhythm of the donor.

In a similar experiment, the odour of the male was found to affect the length of the female cycle. This probably explains why sexually active women tend to have a cycle close to the average length of 29.5 days.

The most interesting feature of the tests was that none of the recipients was aware of any smell coming from the smears. If these odours, operating on an unconscious level, can have such profound effects, it is likely that our lives are influenced in other ways by the human scent.

THE POWER OF THE HUMAN SCENT

Napolean wrote to Josephine from the battlefield 'Ne te lave pas, je reviens.' His request to her not to wash because he was coming reflects the customs of his time. In fact, it was not until the late nineteenth century that body odour came to be considered unpleasant or anti-social. Famous courtesans used to do a roaring trade in handkerchiefs scented with their secretions. This may seem incredible to us today, but our actions would strike them as equally bizarre. Obsessed with personal hygiene, we try to scrub away every trace of human scent, and then add perfumes containing the sexual scents of other animals.

The more expensive perfumes on the market contain animal secretions, such as musk from the ventral pouches of the Himalayan musk deer, castoreum from the beaver's anal gland and civet, scraped from the anal sacs of African cats, while many of the cheaper ones include synthesised forms of these scents. To cap this absurdity, the active ingredient of the most expensive perfume in the world is a secretion which our own bodies manufacture naturally.

The smell chemicals androstenol and androsterone are produced in our saliva, and also in that of pigs. They act as a powerful aphrodisiac on pigs, and synthesised versions of them are sprayed onto sows to make them receptive before artificial insemination. A number of tests have been carried out to find out if these chemicals have a similar effect on us.

Men were shown photographs of women, some of which had been sprayed with androstenol. The photographs scented with the secretion were rated more attractive than those which had not been sprayed. In another study, women who had androstenol applied to their upper lips each day considered themselves to be more submissive than those without it. When the other secretion, androsterone, was sprayed onto a chair in a dentist's waiting room, more women were attracted to sit on it than men.

When people kiss, they exchange not only these secretions in their saliva, but also sebum, which is produced by glands around the mouth after puberty. Some researchers believe that sebum encourages bonding between men and women.

However, none of the tests on any of these secretions is very conclusive. The major problem with investigating the effects of human sexual scents is that many of our actions are dictated by our conscious mind which can moderate or overrule these unconscious influences. This makes our sexual behaviour more complex than that of most other animals, and experimental conditions often exaggerate the difficulty.

For example, vaginal odours, known as copulins, have a strong effect on many mammals, particularly when they indicate that the female is on heat. Yet when men were asked to smell swabs taken from a woman's vagina at different times during the menstrual cycle, they found the smells least attractive at the time of ovulation. However, other mammals are strongly attracted by them which will make it difficult for the perfume manufacturers, who have extracted and patented human copulins, to market them successfully. Polar and grizzly bears are highly responsive to the vaginal scents of menstruating women, and they may even be a factor in bear attacks. In some parts of North America, women are advised not to go camping when they have a period.

It may be that under more natural conditions their effect on men would be very different. Just as the smell of a ripe Camembert is only mouthwatering at the dinner table, the attraction of female odours is likely to depend on their context.

Considering the role of scents in the lives of other animals, it would be suprising if our secretions had no influence at all. Masked as they are by the sexual scents of other animals or the synthesised fragrance of flowers, they probably still affect our behaviour to some extent. It may even be that our exceptionally limited use of the sense of smell, and our twentieth-century obsession with eliminating body odours, are a recognition of the chaos our unmasked scents could create in our overcrowded lives.

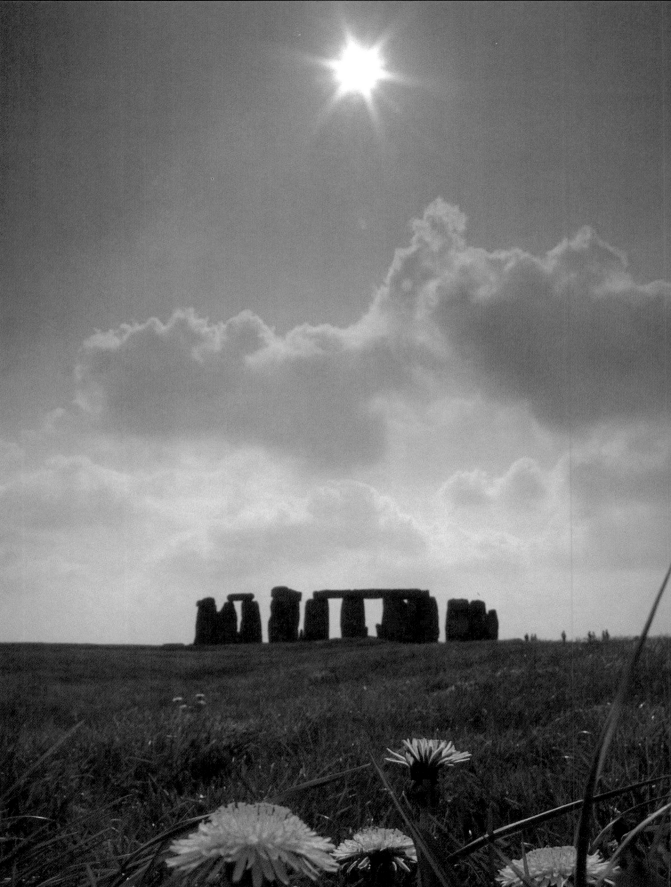

■ SENSE OF TIMING

The solar system has travelled round the galaxy almost 20 times since it was formed, and it has described only a tiny arc of its journey during the two million years that people have been on the Earth. Such vast cosmic movements have little meaning for us, because in comparison our lives are so fleeting. However, early people did study those heavenly cycles which were easily discernible within their lifespan. The daily spin of the Earth, the roughly monthly orbit of the moon, and the yearly passage of the Earth around the sun, were all used to measure the flow of time. Devices, such as sundials, were developed to help keep track of these movements, and their rhythms were recorded and predicted in calendars.

The lives of other creatures span very different periods to our three score years and ten. The oldest known tree was a bristlecone pine in Nevada which lived for 5100 years. To a fly, such an interval would appear infinite, for its life is 85 000 times shorter. Despite this, both creatures sense the passing of time in the same way. The sun is such a powerful influence that its cycle governs all life, whatever its span.

Today, we live in an increasingly artificial environment, and are much less aware of the natural cycles on which we base our system of time. Instead of following the movements of heavenly bodies, we rely on mechanical or electronic clocks to tell the time. However, independently of machines, we do have a natural time sense. We wake and sleep according to the sun's cycle, and research is showing that celestial rhythms still control many other areas of our life.

THE SUN'S CYCLE

The early Earth had little atmosphere to shield it from the searing heart of the sun at mid-day, or the freezing cold of night. Few animals and plants can withstand such extreme temperatures, and the early creatures survived by being active only at certain favourable parts of the day. To enable them to do this, they had to develop a body clock, geared to the sun's cycle. This clock follows a circadian (which means 'about a day') rhythm of approximately 24 hours.

Today, a thick layer of air blankets the Earth, filtering the sun's rays during the day and trapping warmth in at night. But all living things retain a body clock. Every cell in each animal and plant beats to the circadian rhythm. Anyone who has kept a dog or cat will know how accurate this rhythm can be. The errant owner is quickly reminded if a meal or a walk is overdue.

The circadian rhythm is still essential for survival. Each creature has evolved to operate most efficiently during a particular part of the sun's cycle, and some are now locked into their chosen time slot. For example, in many parts of the world, reptiles can only be active during the day. They have little control over their body temperature, and away from the sun's heat they become cool and lethargic. Warm-blooded animals do not have this constraint, although they tend to avoid extremes of temperature.

The daily rising and setting of the sun brings changes not only in temperatures but also in humidity and light. The sun's rays dry up the moisture which amphibians, such as frogs, toads and newts, need. Many of these hide in the day to avoid desiccation, and gather their food during the damper night. The sun's light has the greatest significance for plants, which use it to manufacture their food through photosynthesis. However, many animals have also come to rely on light, particularly those with keen vision. The high speed flight of birds demands good eyesight, and so birds tend to be diurnal. Animals which depend more on other senses can avoid eagle-eyed predators by moving about under cover of darkness. Some animals compromise by being active at dawn and dusk when the hazy twilight helps to hide them.

Above all, operating in different time zones allows animals to exploit their environment to the full. Life exists in all niches on the Earth, from the mountain tops to the bottom of the oceans. Within each niche, similar animals can avoid competing with each other by working shifts. For example, most moths are active during the night, while their relatives, the butterflies, take the day shift, flitting through the warmer, drier hours of sunlight. Some animals have this honed down to a fine art. There are five species of *Dorylus* or driver ants living in the same area of Africa. All move about in huge foraging columns, but each species is active during a different period of the day or night and so they share out their environment over time. Having chosen the shift which suits it best, each animal relies on its circadian rhythm to keep it on schedule.

SETTING THE CLOCK

Although we often try to ignore it, our bodies are also controlled by a circadian rhythm. Being keen-sighted creatures, we are designed to be alert during the day and to sleep through the dark hours. If people are kept awake for long periods of time, their drowsiness lessens in the morning and comes on with increased severity in the evening.

To investigate our rhythms, some individuals have lived for long periods in underground caves, cut off from sunlight. During these experiments the people slept and woke on a regular cycle. However, their 'day' lengthened to nearly 26 hours, so that when they resurfaced, they underestimated the time they had spent below ground.

If any animal or plant is kept in constant artificial light or darkness, its rhythm changes slightly. For some the 'day' grows longer and for others, it shortens. But back in the sunlight, all quickly resume their 24-hour circadian rhythm. The sun seems to act as a master clock, synchronising all the billions of body clocks to its cycle.

Even the simplest organisms have as accurate a body clock as ourselves, sensing light through their cell walls or through special light-sensitive cells. Most plants follow the rhythm of the sun easily, because their leaves act like solar panels, gathering the sun's energy for photosynthesis.

Vertebrates have a special organ, known as the pineal, to detect the daily changes in light. This is situated between the eyes, and in fish, amphibians, reptiles and birds it lies just below the skin, acting as a rudimentary third eye. Indeed, the pineal of a New Zealand reptile known as the tuatara is pigmented and so close to the surface that it looks similar to a real eye. In mammals, the pineal is buried much deeper in the skull. Our eyes detect the light and pass messages to the pineal, which sends the information to our master clock.

The pineal also produces a hormone called melatonin during the hours of darkness, which helps to regulate our cycle. However, the master clock can over-ride the pineal, allowing us to maintain a daily rhythm even in constant light or darkness.

We sometimes disturb this process by moving quickly across time zones on trans-continental flights. Although we can quickly reset our watches, our body clock takes many days to adjust, and so instructs the pineal to produce melatonin at the wrong time of day, causing jet-lag. In the future, it might be possible for us to reset our body clock to the new time zone quickly, by taking a pill containing melatonin at the appropriate time of day.

Problems can also arise for people in urban areas, some of whom suffer from 'winter depression', making them dull and lethargic during the day and unable to sleep at night. This is probably because, locked in the artificial environment of a city in winter, they are exposed to insufficient natural light for their master clock to synchronise its cycle with that of the sun, and so their 'day' grows longer. Such people can be cured by exposure to intense bright light at set times each day which resets their body clock.

In the industrialised world, shift workers may change their sleeping hours every week or even twice a week. Most are able to do this without any marked ill effects. However, night workers will never perform their job as efficiently as they would during the day, for the master clock controls far more than just our cycle of sleeping and waking. This disruption may have more serious consequences than we realise. Flies which have their day length continually varied live a shorter time than those following a more normal routine.

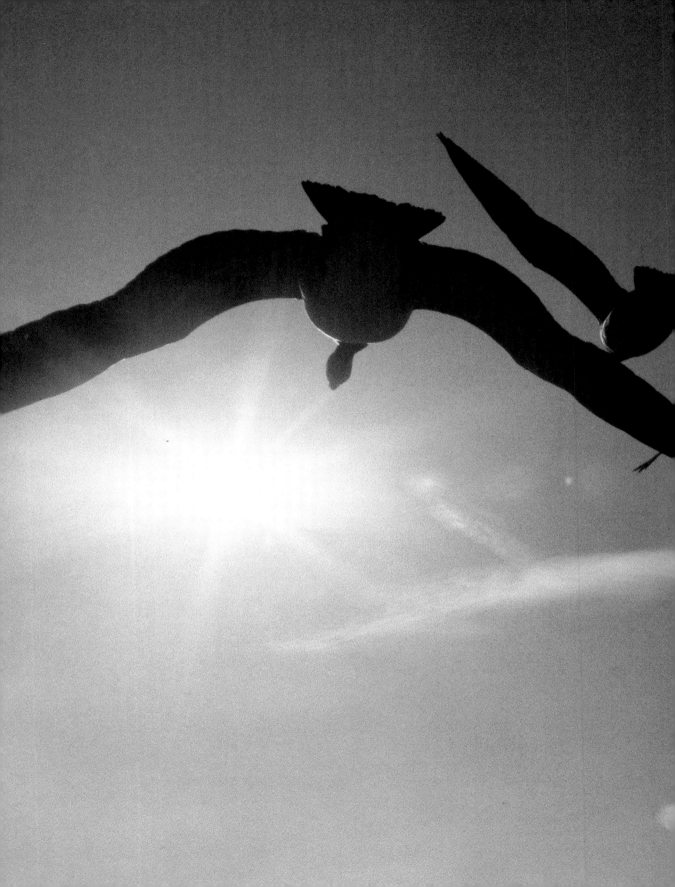

Birds navigate using the sun as a guide to compass direction. To do this they need an accurate internal clock which can compensate for the sun's movement across the sky.

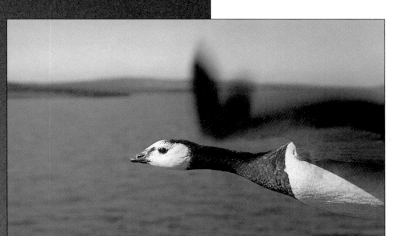

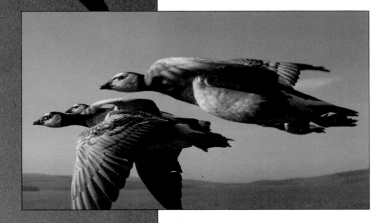

PLANT CLOCKS

At the same time each evening, some house plants, such as mimosa and the prayer plant, fold up their leaves for the night. Many wild plants, including clover and wood sorrel, do the same. If such plants are kept under artificial light these strange movements continue, for they are triggered not by the fading light, but by the plant's biological clock.

The reason for this leaf-folding is a mystery. It may be designed to cut down heat loss from the plant at night. Another theory is that it prevents the leaves from mistaking strong moonlight for the dawn of another day. Such an error could upset the plant's internal clock, causing it to mistime its other activities.

Many plants use their clocks to open and close their flowers at set times each day. The name daisy is derived from 'Day's eye', for this plant opens its flowers at dawn. In some areas, the Goat's Beard is known as 'John-go-to-bed-at-noon' because its flowers close at midday. The dandelion is equally dependable, opening its flowers in the morning and closing them in late afternoon. Its seedheads are actually called 'clocks' in some rural areas. Many plants are so reliable that floral clocks have been designed with flowers arranged round the clock face in the order of their opening and closing times.

Plants open their flowers to lure insect pollinators with their nectar. Even plants which keep their flowers open all the time save energy by only producing nectar at certain periods of the day. So, the insects which feed on nectar need a very well-developed time sense if they are to secure a meal easily.

Some nectar-eating ants cut down on the time they spend searching for food by using their body clock to alert them to meal-times. This gives them an advantage over other insects in their tropical rain forest home. Honeybees show a remarkable ability to synchronise their activities with the opening times of flowers. When tested with a sugar solution resembling nectar, bees were able to distinguish up to nine separate meal times. They were so accurate that frequently bees were ready and waiting when the experimenters arrived to refill the sugar solution. When kept under conditions of constant light and temperature, they still turned up for meals at regular intervals. However, they arrived slightly earlier for each meal, showing that without the regulation of the sun, their 'day' shortens. Like us, bees can also suffer jet-lag. When bees trained to an artificial feeder in Paris were flown to New York, they kept to their established meal times. Only after a few days' exposure to New York sunlight did they readjust to local time.

Normally, of course, bees would not travel such vast distances. However, their daily search for food takes them on journeys requiring considerable navigation skills, and their time sense helps them here as well.

THE SUN COMPASS

When a honeybee finds a new source of food, it senses the direction from the hive to the food using the sun as a compass. It does this by noting the angle the course makes with a point on the horizon directly below the sun, known as the azimuth. However, this point is not a static marker, but moves along the horizon as the sun travels across the sky in an arc. So to maintain a correct course, the bee has to use its body clock to gauge the time and then adjust the angle to compensate for the sun's movement. This is best illustrated in the dance which a successful bee performs on its return to the hive.

The honeybee's dance is very intricate and conveys information about the quality and quantity of the food source as well as its location. It communicates the course by dancing in the appropriate direction on the wall of the hive. Straight up means that the source is in line with the sun, and any other direction indicates the angle of the course away from the sun. As the day progresses, the angle between the food source and the sun alters and the direction given in the bee's dance changes accordingly.

The honeybee shares the ability to use the sun as a compass with a wide range of animals, including ants, sandhoppers, many fish and birds. Most birds use the direction of the sun more than any other navigational aid, and so need a very reliable time sense. Just how accurate they are was demonstrated when some birds were kept under a stationary artificial 'sun'. The birds continued to adjust their bearings as though the sun was moving in its usual arc.

At the appropriate times of the year, caged migrant birds regularly hop in the direction relative to the sun in which they would normally migrate. The apparently magical arrival of migratory birds in the spring and their disappearance in the autumn are just two of the many dramatic events which accompany the climatic variations during the year. These events show that plants and animals have evolved not only a circadian rhythm to regulate their daily lives, but also a way of reliably sensing and responding to the changing seasons.

TIMING THE SEASONS

The seasons occur because the spinning Earth is tilted on its axis relative to the sun. So, as our planet moves on its yearly orbit around the sun, the northern hemisphere is angled towards the sun for part of the year, and the southern hemisphere is tilted towards it for the other part. The effects of this are most extreme at the poles, which are bathed in light for up to 24 hours a day over a short summer, and then plunged into twilight darkening to permanent night during the long polar winter.

At lower latitudes, the hours of daylight increase up to mid-summer but never obliterate the night, while sunlight penetrates even in the middle of winter. In these

◼ FLORAL CLOCK

◼ Carl Linnaeus, the 18th-century botanist, arranged flowers in a sequence so that their opening and closing times could be used to tell the time. Such floral clocks rely on the fact that the flower's petal movements are predictable from day to day. The petal movements are controlled by a circadian rhythm or the plant's sensitivity to light. Bees and other pollinators soon learn to synchronise their activity to these flowers, arriving only when the blooms are open and secreting nectar. Floral clocks are only accurate over a limited area, for the opening times vary with geographical position and altitude.

STAR OF BETHLEHEM (OPENS)

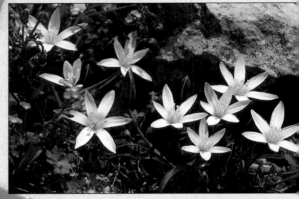

COMMON NIPPLEWORT (CLOSE

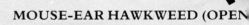

FIELD MARIGOLD (OPENS)

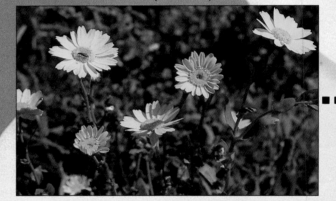

MOUSE-EAR HAWKWEED (OPEN

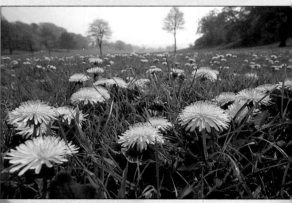

DANDELION (OPENS)

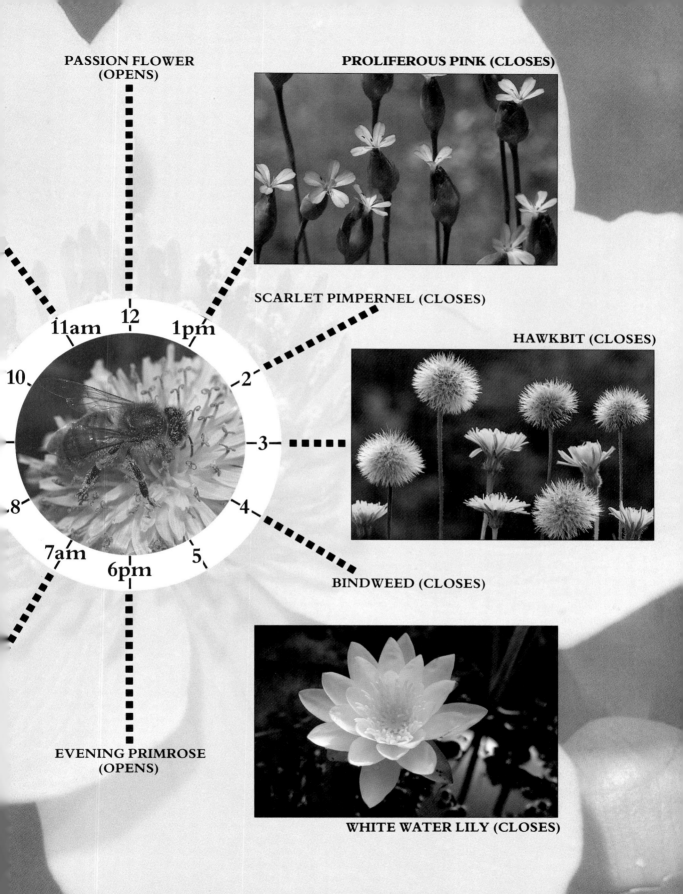

PASSION FLOWER (OPENS)

PROLIFEROUS PINK (CLOSES)

SCARLET PIMPERNEL (CLOSES)

HAWKBIT (CLOSES)

BINDWEED (CLOSES)

EVENING PRIMROSE (OPENS)

WHITE WATER LILY (CLOSES)

11am 12 1pm 2 3 4 5 6pm 7am 8 10

latitudes two additional seasons – spring and autumn – mark the passing of the year. The variation in day length decreases with distance from the poles and vanishes at the Equator, which receives 12 hours of light each day throughout the year.

The areas of the world tilted away from the sun not only receive fewer hours of daylight but also less heat during those hours. The sun's rays have to travel through more of the Earth's absorbent atmosphere to reach these areas than they do when the sun is overhead, resulting in a drop in temperature as winter approaches. This is a problem for plants because they already have fewer daylight hours in which to manufacture their food, and cannot grow at all if the temperature falls below 6 degrees Celsius.

In the tropics, plants receive enough light and heat all year round, but they also need water, and seasonal variations in rainfall affect their productivity. Since animals depend either directly or indirectly on plants for food, all life is affected by the variations in weather over the seasons. As a result, animals and plants have had to find ways of both coping with and predicting these seasonal changes.

Detecting the seasons is not as easy as it may appear, because the weather does not vary reliably. Frosts can occur well into summer, while snow may fall in spring, and autumn days can be as balmy as summer or bitter as winter. So the spring flowers which bloom at the same time each year, and the swifts and swallows which return so precisely to their nest sites, are clearly responding to a more dependable guide. The answer may seem obvious now, but it was not realised until the 1920s that creatures sense variations in the length of the day.

Of all the changes caused by the Earth's tilt, the variations in day length follow the smoothest and most regular pattern. Animals and plants respond to these changes through a process known as photoperiodism.

PLANT CALENDARS

A plant's leaves are ideally placed to detect day length, for they are designed to pick up the sun's light for photosynthesis. The green colour of the leaf is due to a substance called chlorophyll which also contains the pigment phytochrome. This pigment is sensitive to red light and changes to a different form when the red part of the sun's light hits it, reverting back again when night falls. The relative concentrations of these two forms of phytochrome can influence many aspects of the plant's life, including the formation of roots, the colour of leaves, and flowering.

Some, such as carnations, radishes, scarlet pimpernels and clover, flower in the spring when the days are lengthening, and so are called long-day plants. Chrysanthemums, poinsettia, corn, coffee and others flower during the shortening days of autumn and are known as short-day plants. There are also many which flower at any time regardless of day length, and these include dandelions, sunflowers, tomatoes and potatoes.

Despite the terms 'short-day' and 'long-day', the cue which these plants are following is actually the length of the night. Using artificial light to break up a long night into two short ones promotes the flowering of long-day plants and hinders the flowering of short-day ones. Market gardeners often use artificial light and dark cloths to adjust the length of the night and so persuade plants to flower at unnatural times of the year.

Many plants need a period of dormancy before they leaf and flower and the timing of this period is often influenced by the temperature. The spreading leaf canopy of trees in the spring is initiated partly by temperature. However, the most striking change in the life of deciduous trees – the golden spectacle of the autumn – is controlled almost completely by day length.

Although there may be heavy rainfall during the winter, a deciduous tree's roots cannot absorb water from the cold soil as quickly as water evaporates from its leaves. So such trees have to lose their leaves in the autumn to prevent water loss. They rely on day length to trigger the shedding because the process is a complex one. If the trees waited for the onset of cold weather before starting to shed, they could be damaged by the shortfall in water by the time the process was complete.

A tree cannot simply drop its leaves because it would be discarding vast quantities of nutrients. So it first absorbs the sugars, protein, minerals and chlorophyll in the leaves. The removal of the green chlorophyll unmasks the red, gold and brown pigments which leaves also contain, creating the beautiful hues of autumn. Once the nutrients are absorbed, a hormone initiates the destruction of a band of cells at the base of each leaf. This weakens the leaf's connection to the tree so much that even a light breeze can blow it off. Because day length controls this process, trees in cities illuminated by street lights tend to lose their leaves later than their rural relatives.

Animals also need to cope with the severity of winter, and they have developed a variety of ways of doing this.

ANIMALS IN WINTER

The onset of winter presents most animals with the dual problem of keeping warm and finding enough to eat. Some mammals grow a thicker coat of fur so that they retain more of their body heat. Those which live in areas regularly covered in snow may also change the colour of their fur to white. This camouflage is adopted by the arctic hare and stoat, and their transformation is controlled by the shortening days of autumn.

This same cue also seems to trigger a decrease in growth and even appetite among mammals such as deer, sheep and goats. When red deer were supplied with plenty of food all year round, they ate much more in the summer than in the winter. A young red deer puts on weight at a considerable rate during its first summer, but its growth

■ DAYLENGTH AND THE SEASONS

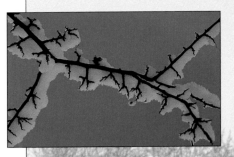

■ **Spring** Spring flowers *(below)* are triggered into bloom by a combination of rising temperatures and lengthening days, detected through the leaves.

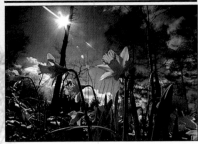

■ Each year the temperate regions of the world experience a seemingly miraculous succession of natural events, all timed with unerring precision. The synchroniser for much of this activity is the change in the number of daylight hours as the earth tilts on its axis (represented by the central, light portion of the main picture). These changes are more dependable than those of temperature and so many animals and plants rely on them to time their lives.

Winter With much of the ground, and even trees *(above)* covered in snow during the shortening days of winter, some animals *(below)* hibernate to avoid the harsh conditions. An internal clock will wake them in spring.

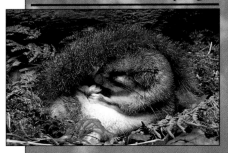

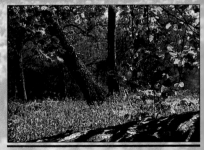

■ **Spring** Bluebells *(above)* race to beat the opening of the leaf canopy, which is also triggered by the lengthening days.

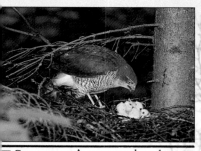

Summer A sparrowhawk on the nest *(above)*. The reproductive cycle of birds is controlled by daylength detected by a pineal organ directly under the skull.

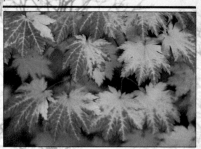

Autumn The shortening days of autumn trigger the spectacular colour changes of the leaves *(below)*.

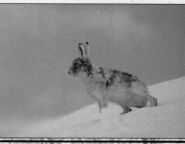

Winter The camouflage coat of the Arctic hare *(above)*, and other mammals such as the stoat and Arctic fox, are caused by the shortening days of winter.

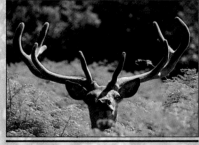

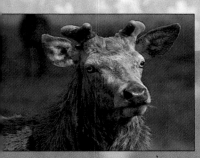

Summer/Autumn The growth of deer antlers in late spring and through the summer months *(left)* is the result of hormone changes initiated by changing daylength and sensed through the eyes. Later in the year, the short days of autumn also stimulate sexual activity *(above)*. This ensures that the young are not born until the following spring and so avoid the harsh winter.

Winter In the dormant months of winter, tree buds await the lengthening days that signal the arrival of spring *(below)*.

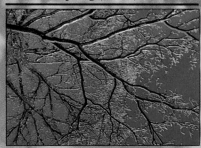

is reduced to less than half of this rate during the winter. The decrease is not simply a result of its reduced appetite. Even if these animals eat the same restricted amount every day, they still grow more rapidly in the summer than in the winter. This makes very good sense, for in the wild there is much less food available during the winter, and the plants which can be found are less nutritious in winter than in summer.

Experiments have indicated that these changes are induced by day length. Mammals keep track of this using the pineal gland which also regulates their bodies' circadian rhythm. In the day the pineal creates and stores a chemical called seratonin, and during the night this is converted into melatonin and released into the bloodstream. As the night lengthens, the production time of melatonin increases, and this appears to stimulate the production of hormones which transform the appetite, metabolic rate, and colour and growth of fur.

Other animals avoid the difficulties of winter by reducing their metabolic rate even further and going into a state of torpor or hibernating. When in torpor, an animal's body temperature drops slightly, and its heartbeat and breathing rates are reduced. Bears, squirrels and badgers are some of the many animals which overwinter in this way.

In hibernating animals, the body temperature falls much further, to just above freezing, while heartbeat and all the other bodily functions slow down to a barely perceptible pace. Animals which hibernate include hedgehogs, ground squirrels, dormice, bats, hamsters and one bird. The poorwill is a North American nightjar which for much of the year catches insects through the twilight hours of dawn and dusk. If bad weather prevented it from hunting at these times it would starve. The poorwill evades this risk by hibernating in the crevice of a rock wall, which it returns to year after year.

The ground squirrel is a much more typical hibernator. Over the summer it builds up a surplus of fat and as autumn draws on it returns to an underground burrow. There it has a store of food and a nest of grass and other materials in which it curls up into a ball, tucking in extremities. Its temperature falls each night until it reaches 5 degrees Celsius and the animal then becomes dormant. Every four weeks the body temperature rises and the ground squirrel awakens and moves about, even venturing outside the burrow. However, for most of the winter it remains still and cold, giving every appearance of being dead. Although hibernation can be dangerous and some creatures never awaken from it, it is less lethal to the animals which opt for it than the rigours of a harsh winter would be. They are prompted to hibernate by a drop in temperature, but this cue only works if the days are also shortening.

Hibernating animals need to awaken on schedule so that they can mate and have their young while food is plentiful. Once dormant, however, their metabolism slows down so much that the pineal is virtually switched off, and how they manage to rouse themselves at the correct time remains a mystery. It raises the possibility that their master clock can continue to keep track of the passage of time even when all bodily functions are drastically reduced.

BREEDING ON CUE

Most mammals have their young in the spring when plant growth is at its maximum, insects are plentiful and the weather is mild. To achieve this, larger mammals, such as goats, sheep and deer, must mate in the shortening days of autumn because they have a gestation period of about six months. Smaller mammals, such as cats, rabbits and ferrets, have only a short gestation and so can mate in the lengthening days that signal the end of winter. The cue to start the reproductive cycle is, again, the variation in day length. Deer and sheep can be induced to mate by artificially shortening the days, while lengthening the days has the same effect on ferrets.

The appropriate change in day length causes the animals' bodies to produce hormones which activate their reproductive organs. This system can present difficulties for animals which spend much of their life underground. At least one, the hamster, has found a simple solution. It comes to the surface for a few seconds several times each day, and two short exposures to light separated by 12 hours are enough to initiate its reproductive cycle.

The single cue of day length triggers the breeding of a host of other animals. For centuries, the Japanese have induced captive birds to sing their courtship songs out of season by using artificial light to lengthen the days, a method known as 'yogai'.

Similarly, it has long been known that hens lay more eggs if they are kept under artificial illumination. The sexual organs of birds enlarge dramatically as the days lengthen and then shrivel up again after breeding.

In the tropics, where day length varies only slightly, birds tend to use other guides, particularly rainfall. However, even some tropical species, such as quelea finches, can be persuaded to breed by artificially adjusting the day length.

Birds show the greatest sensitivity to day length of any vertebrates. This cue prompts not only breeding, but also their annual moult, and the vast journeys of migrating birds. Reptiles are also strongly affected by the photoperiod, and even some fish use it.

In the darkness of the ocean depths, the varying light of the seasons goes unnoticed but many shallow-water fish respond to it. Tropical aquarium favourites, such as guppies and swordtails, start to breed as soon as the days lengthen, while the sexual organs of the goldfish degenerate if it is kept in the dark. Trout are also sensitive to the photoperiod, and farmers of trout sometimes induce young fish to breed early by artificially lengthening the days.

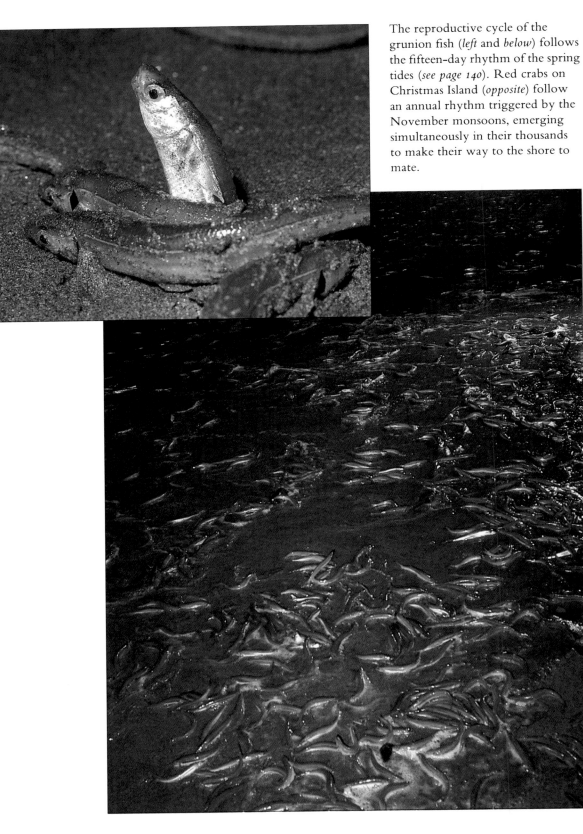

The reproductive cycle of the grunion fish (*left* and *below*) follows the fifteen-day rhythm of the spring tides (*see page 140*). Red crabs on Christmas Island (*opposite*) follow an annual rhythm triggered by the November monsoons, emerging simultaneously in their thousands to make their way to the shore to mate.

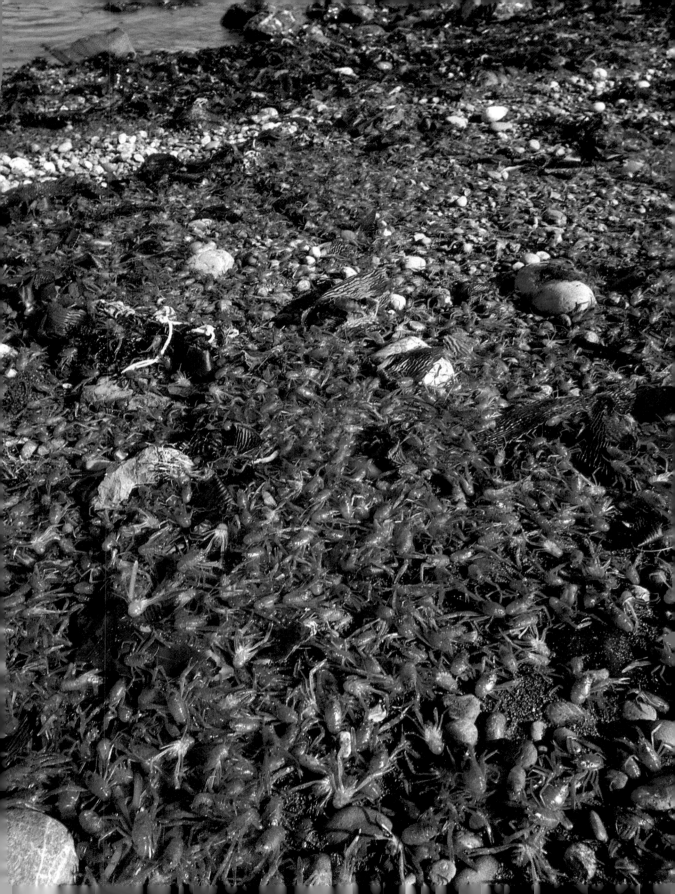

Even some invertebrates, such as insects and snails, time their breeding by the photoperiod. With such a huge range of reproductive activity stimulated by the sun, it might be thought that no other trigger was needed. However, another heavenly body – the moon – has an equally dramatic effect on the sex life of many animals.

LUNAR RHYTHMS

Moonbeams are not the moon's own light, but the sun's rays reflected off the side of the moon facing the sun. As the moon orbits the Earth, we see varying amounts of its illuminated face. When the moon lies between us and the sun, its light side is hidden, and we call this phase a new moon. As the moon moves round, part of its illuminated face becomes visible, first as a crescent and then swelling through a half moon into a gibbous shape. Halfway round its orbit, the moon is lying on the opposite side of the Earth to the sun, and we see a full moon, with all of its light side in view. As the moon completes its orbit it seems to shrink or wane through the phases of gibbous, half moon and cresent, back to new moon. The whole cycle takes 29.5 days, and each phase occurs with absolute regularity.

Ancient people revered the moon, and followed its movements closely, holding festivals and rites at particular phases of the moon. They associated it particularly with fertility, and modern research is revealing that the moon does influence the reproductive cycles of at least some creatures.

For centuries, fishermen have maintained that the size of their catch is affected by the phases of the moon. Some investigations into herring and eel catches have suggested that there is a link, probably because the activities of these fish vary according to the amount of light at night. Another fisherman's tale, common in the Mediterranean, is that sea urchins taste best around the full moon. This would be the case if sea urchins produce eggs at this time. One species, which lives in a small area round the Suez, certainly does ripen its eggs at full moon, and a sea urchin off California has a similar lunar cycle, so there may be some substance to the fishermen's claim.

However, the clearest example of the power of the moon is a strange event which occurs in the seas round Fiji and Samoa each November. At full moon the sea turns a milky white colour and provides the local fishermen with a free harvest of highly nutritious protein. This apparently magical gift is actually provided by the palolo, a tropical relative of the lugworm, which lives in crevices in coral. As November approaches, the end part of its body starts to swell until, on the night of the full moon, it breaks off and explodes, releasing eggs or sperm. By using the moon to time their breeding, the palolo worms ensure that they all spawn simultaneously. This greatly increases the chances of survival of the young, for the fishermen and the many marine predators combined can only harvest a small proportion of this vast feast.

Very recently an even more spectacular occurrence was discovered, which is probably the world's greatest synchronised natural event. The Great Barrier Reef, which hugs the north-east shore of Australia for 2000 kilometres, owes its existence to millions of tiny animals called coral polyps. The Reef is built up from the hard skeletons of dead polyps, and forms a base for the living coral. Permanently attached to their stony home, the living polyps reproduce sexually by releasing eggs or sperm into the sea. The timing of their reproduction is linked to temperature, and to a phase of the moon. In this way, the polyps synchronise the release of their sexual cells so precisely that the event occurs at the same hour on a particular night each year, turning the sea into a multi-coloured reproductive soup.

Many marine organisms time their reproduction by the moon, and some land organisms also breed by the lunar cycle, particularly those living in equatorial regions where day length is virtually constant and so cannot be used as a guide. In Lake Victoria in Uganda, the aquatic larvae of a mayfly emerge and become adults two days after the full moon. These adults subsequently lay eggs which follow the same cycle. Away from the Equator, the mayfly's breeding loses its lunar rhythm. The sooty terns of the tropical Ascension Islands also seem to use the moon to synchronise breeding for they all return to the islands to nest every tenth lunar month. In fact, so many animals respond to a lunar cycle that people have wondered whether the ancients were right to associate the moon with human fertility.

The only human sexual rhythm is the female menstrual cycle, and this lasts, on average, one lunar cycle. In addition, our average gestation period is exactly nine lunar cycles. Hospital records show no link between the timing of births and the phases of the moon. However, in our modern industrial world, few women have sufficient exposure to moonlight to be able to synchronise with the lunar rhythm. When women were given artificial moonlight for three consecutive nights once a month, their cycles became synchronised to the lunar rhythm. So in the past, when we were not shielded from moonlight, it may have had an effect.

The moon causes another rhythm, which has little influence on us but is of profound importance to life along the shore, and that is the rhythm of the tides.

TIMING THE TIDES

Just as the Earth's gravitational force keeps the moon in orbit, so the moon exerts a force on the Earth. This pull has little effect on the land but is strong enough to move the waters. It causes the sea beneath the moon to bulge towards it, while the water on the opposite side of the Earth bulges away. As the Earth spins, the two bulges move round, creating the twice daily rhythm of the tides. The moon moves in the same direction as the Earth's rotation, slightly extending the interval between high tides to 12.4 hours.

The tidal rhythm makes the shoreline one of the harshest environments in the world. For part of the day it is pounded by water and for the rest of the time it is exposed to the desiccating heat of the sun or the bitter cold of night. The creatures which live there manage to survive by being able to predict these violent changes.

Golden brown algae, known as diatoms, live in the sands on the north shore of Cape Cod. Each day at low tide these extraordinary microscopic plants glide up through the sand to soak up the sun's energy for photosynthesis. There are so many of these tiny organisms that they form a vast golden carpet along the shoreline. Then, just before the tide returns, the carpet vanishes. As if obeying some universal command, the diatoms move simultaneously back into the sand. If these plants are kept in a laboratory, they act in exactly the same way. Diatoms, along with many other marine organisms, have an accurate body clock tuned to the rhythm of the tides. As with the circadian rhythm, under constant conditions the tidal rhythm continues but its length changes slightly.

On the shores of Brittany live flatworms which behave very similarly to the diatoms. This is because they share their bodies with algae and have to bring the algae to the surface at low tides so that they can manufacture food. In return for providing a protected home and transport, the flatworms receive some of this food.

The fiddler crabs of North America emerge from their burrows at low tide to scavenge for food. The males may also battle with each other, and try to entice females back to their burrows with beckoning movements of an extra-large claw. All this activity suddenly ceases and they scuttle back into their burrows before the tide washes in. Shore crabs, which live higher up the beach, time their activities to coincide with the high tide. This enables them to forage under cover of water, hidden from predatory birds.

The 12.4-hour rhythm is not the only tidal cycle that marine life responds to. The sun also exerts a force on the Earth, but because it is so much further away, its pull is only one quarter of that of the moon. When the sun and moon are at right angles to the Earth, as at each half moon, their pulls counteract each other, producing the weak neap tides. However, when they are in line with the Earth, at full and new moons, their forces combine to create the strong spring tides.

The approximately fifteen-day rhythm of spring and neap tides is of vital importance to some creatures. Once every fifteen days, during the strong spring tides, areas normally immersed in water are briefly exposed to the air. An aquatic midge, known as *Clunio,* lives among seaweed in one such area. This remarkable insect manages to time its reproductive cycle to coincide with its short period of exposure. As soon as the tide goes out, it emerges from its pupal case, mates, and lays its eggs before the tide returns. The adults have only two hours to complete their life cycle, and the males actually help the females out of their pupal cases to speed up mating.

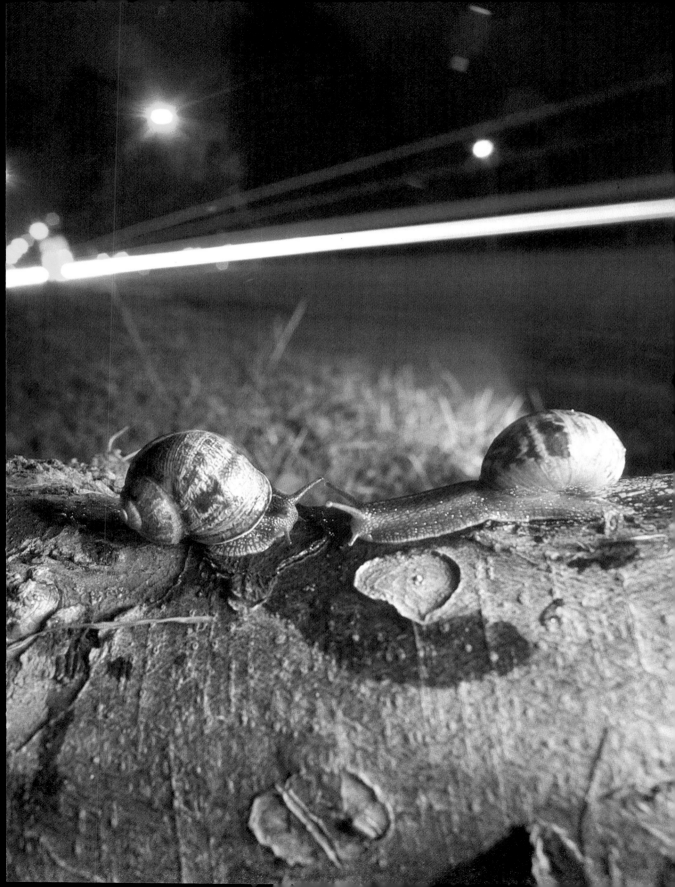

The midge's body clock keeps track of the fifteen-day rhythm of spring tides. In the southern part of its range, it synchronises its clock to the phases of the moon, but in the north, where nights are frequently overcast, the tide itself acts as the regulator.

The grunion fish of California have an equally strange reproductive ritual. Every fifteen days, when the spring tides are at their peak, vast numbers of grunion ride in on the crests of waves and deliberately strand themselves on the shore. The females bury their tails in the sand and each lays a stream of eggs, while the males, entwined around the females, fertilise the eggs. The fish then propel themselves back to catch the next wave. The eggs remain in the damp sand, safe from marine predators, until they hatch out fifteen days later and swim off on the next high spring tide.

Such fifteen-day cycles are quite unusual, but many creatures can measure a much longer interval.

CLOCKING UP THE YEARS

When European trees were taken to the tropics to grace the residences of nineteenth-century colonists, they continued to grow and shed their leaves at regular intervals. However, in their natural laboratory of unchanging day length, the trees' 'year' gradually took up a period slightly different from a true year. This was the first clear demonstration that organisms can possess a yearly or circannual rhythm, regulated by day length.

A yearly body clock is of most significance in the tropics, where there are few seasonal indicators to alert animals and plants to the passing of the year. Many birds which overwinter in equatorial regions rely on a circannual rhythm to time their departure. When warblers were kept under constant lighting conditions, they continued to become restless at the times when they would normally migrate. However, such time-keeping pales into insignificance beside the ability of some creatures, which can actually clock up the years and lock into much longer periods.

Once every 120 years, Chinese umbrella bamboos all over the world simultaneously burst into flower, spread their seed, and then die. Many other species of bamboo also synchronise their flowering, although they use different intervals, such as 10, 20 and 90 years.

Equally eccentric are the periodic cicadas of the United States. These insects spend years underground as larvae, sucking the sap from the roots of trees. Then, on some mysterious cue, they emerge simultaneously from the soil and change into winged adults. Within three weeks they die, having laid the eggs of the next generation which will be in the soil until the time comes to repeat the cycle.

The periodic swarming mass of adults provides such a surfeit for predators that the majority of the cicadas survive to lay eggs. The various species of cicada differ in the length of the life cycle but, interestingly, the interval between egg and adult is always a prime number – 13 or 17 years. This makes it very difficult for predators to multiply their numbers in order to make the most of these periodic gluts.

To be able to synchronise their emergence the cicadas must have an inbuilt timer which can count the passing years even though the animals are buried under the soil. Many insects time the much shorter periods they spend resting over winter as eggs or pupae during a phase known as diapause. Similarly, hibernating mammals can accurately time their awakening.

These animals perceive time very differently during their resting and active phases. A hibernator's metabolism slows down so much when it becomes dormant that time appears to speed by and the winter is over in a trice. Even when active, a time interval does not seem the same to a cicada as to a ground squirrel or to ourselves.

TIME PERCEPTION

The bristlecone pine's life span is more than 70 times longer than ours. We, in our turn, live 70 times longer than the smallest mammal, the shrew, and 1200 times longer than a fly. However, these creatures do not perceive their time on Earth in the same way. The three weeks of a fly's life appear much longer to the fly than they do to us. Although we both have circadian rhythms which divide our time up into days, the fly lives its day at a much faster pace than we do.

Anyone who has tried to swat a fly will know that its reactions are almost instantaneous. Its eyes can discern very small intervals of time (it can respond to a falling hand in less than one hundredth of a second), and our clumsy attempts to kill it must appear ponderously slow, as if filmed in slow motion. The cockroach has a similarly high-speed existence and can react to any attempt to crush it in a fiftieth of a second, while our own reaction time is a tenth of a second.

Birds can also detect much smaller intervals of time than us. Birds' songs often sound varied and melodious to us, but if they are recorded and played back at slow speed, they are found to have vastly more detail than we realise. If noises are separated by very short intervals we hear them as a continous sound. Many birds, on the other hand, hear as separate sounds noises which are separated by an interval of two microseconds or less. One of the most remarkable examples of this is the duet of the African bou-bou shrike, in which each of the pair sings alternately. The time interval between one bird stopping and the other starting is so short that we cannot detect it, and the duet sounds to us like a continuous solo.

In contrast the world appears to move at an incredibly fast pace to a snail. If a snail is tapped on the head with a stick, it quickly withdraws into its shell. However, if the frequency of the taps is increased to four a second, its behaviour changes and it tries to

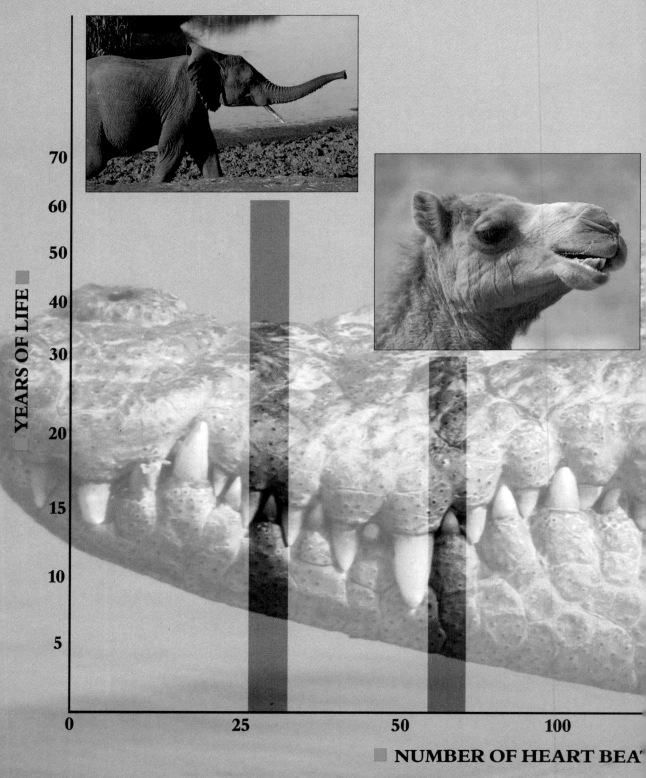

RATES OF LIVING

YEARS OF LIFE

NUMBER OF HEART BEAT

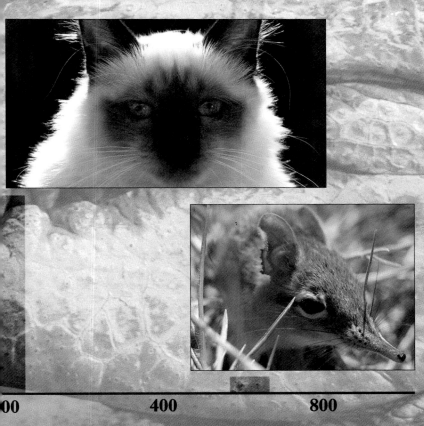

As heartbeat rates are linked to breathing and other physiological processes, they can be used to indicate the rate at which an animal lives its life. All mammals that reach old age have approximately the same number of heartbeats in their lives, so if the heartbeat rate for various animals is plotted against their length of life the result is a graph that follows a straight line.

Heartbeat rate is also governed by the size of the animal: the heart of a small animal, such as an elephant shrew, beats approximately 25 times faster than that of an elephant, and so the animal has a correspondingly shorter life. Fortunately we are exceptions to this: according to our size we should die at about 25 years, but for some reason not yet fully understood, animals with large brains tend to live longer.

Reptiles, too, are exceptions to the rule, for their rate of living also varies with temperature. A crocodile's heart rate may be 70 beats per minute when the animal is warm and drop below 30 beats per minute when cold. As a result, many reptiles are long-lived animals.

00   400   800

ACH MINUTE

crawl onto the stick. The reason for this is that the snail can only perceive events which are more than one quarter of a second apart, so a stick which is moved four times a second appears to be stationary. In comparison with birds and even with ourselves, this animal really does live its life at a snail's pace.

For those animals which have backbones, the rate of their heartbeats is a very good indication of the rate at which they live their lives. Each animal breathes about once every 3.9 heartbeats, and other bodily functions are similarly linked to the rate of the heart. Remarkably, most animals that reach old age have each had, on average, the same number of heartbeats in their life. The allotted number for each heart is about 800 million.

An animal's pace of life is known as its rate of physiological time to distinguish it from the natural rhythms of time which all animals share. The physiological time of cold-blooded animals, such as reptiles and amphibians, varies with the temperature. In birds and mammals, the rate of physiological time depends on body size.

Small mammals tend to have rapid heartbeats and a fast metabolic rate giving them a high-speed life, while for large mammals the reverse is true. For example, the smallest mammal, the shrew, lives its life about 30 times faster than the elephant. To the shrew, 24 hours seems so long that it divides it up into many smaller intervals of activity and rest, effectively experiencing many days within one rotation of the Earth. The shrew's heart beats almost 1000 times a minute, while the elephant uses up only 30 during the same period. Their lifespans show a corresponding difference. Few shrews live as long as 1.5 years, while many elephants plod along for over 50 years.

We are fortunate in being an exception to these rules. According to our size, we should die at about 25 years, by which age we should also have run out of heartbeats, having used up well over 800 million. For a reason not fully understood, animals with large brains have extended natural lifespans. However, along with other animals our perception of time changes as we age.

HUMAN TIME

We are all familiar with the fact that the days of our childhood seemed to stretch out, passing more and more quickly as we grew. One reason for this is that our metabolic rate slows down as we age. At birth, the heart races along at 140 beats a minute, but by the time we reach adulthood the rate has dropped to 70 beats a minute. These changes in metabolic rate affect our rate of physiological time, although they cannot account for all the changes in time perception we experience as we age.

The body of a young child works at the maximum rate, enabling the child to process far more information in a given time than an adult could. A child is also much more stimulated by everything it perceives because the world is new and exciting. For elderly people, time speeds by, partly because their metabolic rate has slowed down but also because life holds far fewer surprises for them.

Our time perception can be altered in other ways. To someone with a high fever, time passes slowly. The same effect can be brought about by drugs such as amphetamines, cannabis and even coffee. Barbiturates and alcohol have the opposite effect, allowing time to slip by unnoticed.

Some of these shifts in time perception are due to changes in metabolic rate produced by fever and drugs, but the mind also plays a part. The two factors working together are most apparent when we experience a sudden shock. The hormone adrenalin pours into the bloodstream, raising the heartbeat and metabolic rate. At the same time, the rate at which information is processed by the brain increases dramatically, making us better able to deal with an emergency. This makes time appear to slow down so that we remember the details of an accident, such as a car crash, as though it occurred in slow motion.

In the natural world, the same shift in time perception probably occurs whenever a predator encounters a prey. However, as with all the senses, we can only guess at how other creatures perceive the world. We can assess what information each animal receives, but its brain may interpret and remember this information in many different ways. It is this influence of the mind which ultimately gives each animal its unique view of the world.

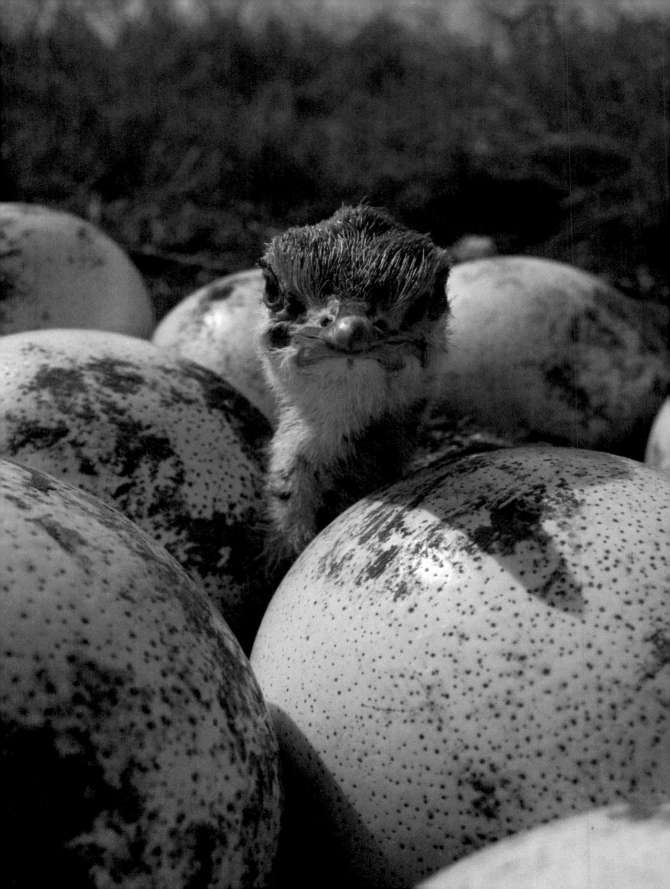

■ MAKING SENSE

We are primarily visual animals, and so may be unaware of how important a part our other senses play in our lives until one of them is lost. When people are deprived of hearing they immediately feel isolated. Not only are they cut off from our main channel of communication, but they are unable to detect danger signals, such as the sound of approaching traffic. Most of us have experienced the temporary loss of smell and taste caused by a heavy cold. Today this simply impairs our enjoyment of shop-bought food, but in the past any inability to discriminate between poisonous and edible wild plants could have had serious consequences. Similarly, many people have had their sense of touch removed temporarily over a small area by a dentist's anaesthetic. While the numbness continues, the mouth can be scalded, bitten or cut without the person realising it.

So, each of our senses aids survival in some way, and each contributes to our awareness of the environment. All animals view the world through a combination of senses. As we have seen, the stimuli that an animal responds to, and their relative importance, vary from species to species, giving each animal slightly different information about the world. However, an animal's perception is not necessarily dependent solely on the stimuli detected by its sense organs. The information received passes to the brain, where it is analysed and may be altered. The brain's modifications are based on the knowledge the animal has accumulated during its life, a process which can commence even before birth.

FIRST PERCEPTIONS

A mammal embryo's senses begin to stir while it is still in the womb. A sense of touch arises first in the area that will become the nose and mouth, and this allows the embryo to detect whether it is resting comfortably. Then the embryo starts to respond to gravity, as the system of semi-circular canals forms in the developing ear, and it is able to orient itself correctly in the womb.

Shortly afterwards, the ear becomes capable of hearing. Initially, the embryo's sound world is dominated by the reassuring heartbeats of its mother. Soon it can also pick up noises from the outside world, although these have to pass through the mother's body and so are muffled. At this stage, the embryo can hear only low frequencies, for its sensitivity to high frequencies does not develop until just before birth.

The growing embryo experiences the circadian rhythm of its mother's body temperature and blood pressure, as well as her cycle of activity and sleep. So its master clock is able to synchronise with her 24-hour rhythm, and the embryonic clock may decide the timing of the birth.

Like mammal embryos, young birds are able to eavesdrop on the world from inside the egg. The chicks of many ground-nesting birds, such as quail, can even communicate from egg to egg. Their faint cheeps and clicks help the chicks to synchronise hatching so that the brood can follow their mother soon after birth. The embryonic chicks can also hear their parents' calls and instinctively fall silent when the adult gives an alarm cry.

As well as having instinctive responses, the young of some communal nesting birds, such as guillemots, start learning sounds while still in the egg. After hatching, these chicks are able to recognise their parents by their calls. Most birds cannot identify their parents at birth and simply follow the first moving object they see. This system is fairly infallible in the wild because a parent never strays far from its brood. In captivity, however, a newly hatched chick may become confused and adopt another animal, a human, or even a ball, as its 'parent'.

The young of deer, antelope and other mammals at risk from predators, emerge into the world with very well-developed eyes. Mammals which are born in protected nests, such as cats and mice, do not open their eyes for several days. Even then their sight does not function fully, and unless they use their eyes, and so form critical connections between the eyes and the brain, their vision is impaired permanently. The importance of this formative stage was shown by kittens brought up in a room decorated with black and white vertical stripes. When the kittens had to view the real world, they were unable to perceive any horizontal structures.

Like birds, many young mammals instinctively follow any large moving object, until their senses are sufficiently developed to allow them to recognise individuals. In mammals, however, smell is often as important as vision for imprinting.

An animal's search for food is also instinctive initially, becoming more refined as the information from their sense organs is aided by experience. When young horses and deer first try to suckle, they reach upwards and sideways for any protrusion, often spending a considerable time searching fruitlessly under their mother's forelegs. Once they have located a nipple, however, they can return to it effortlessly. Similarly, newly hatched waterfowl and pheasant chicks instinctively peck at any green spot. Within a short time they have learnt to recognise the items in their diet and can feed independently.

As a young animal's knowledge grows, its mind plays an increasing role in interpreting the information provided by stimuli. The clearest example of this is the way an animal learns to recognise features in its immediate environment and builds up a mental map of its home range.

MENTAL MAPS

When a young animal first explores its home area, its brain receives an overwhelming array of new sensory data. After several journeys, information about the more permanent features of its surroundings has been stored. Soon the animal has built up a mental map of its range and knows the relative position of features and the quickest route between them. Then any alteration or addition to the environment can be quickly detected and investigated.

In the same way, when we move into a new area, our only point of reference is usually the new home. Within a short time we have become familiar with visual features such as shops, churches and unusual buildings, and can find our way around with ease. Like us, many animals rely heavily on vision to create their mental maps.

When the tide is in, the frill-finned goby explores the rocky bed of its shore home. As the tide recedes, most shore life is left stranded in rock pools. By consulting its mental map, however, the goby can locate all the pools and leap unerringly between them. Similarly, the digger wasp stores visual details of its sandy home. It builds tunnels in the sand and stocks them with caterpillars to feed to its grubs. The insect is able to locate its larders by memorising the position of nearby stones or twigs. If these features are rearranged, the wasp has great difficulty in finding its food stocks.

The rat uses smell as well as vision to build up mental maps of its regular routes. These may become so ingrained that it will continue to leap over the position of a remembered obstacle after the obstruction has been removed. This apparently mindless behaviour saves the rat valuable thinking time when being chased by a predator.

Mental maps are particularly useful for animals, such as owls, which are active at times when sensory data may be very limited. On some nights there is insufficient light to provide a clear view for even the owl's supersensitive eyes. By keeping to familiar territory, the owl can fly at speed through dense woodland, relying on its mental map to fill in missing details.

As well as covering the home range, our mental maps often include mountains or tall buildings which we have never visited but which we use as reference points. The range of the landmarks we can observe, however, is limited by the fact that our eyes are less than 2 metres off the ground. Birds commonly fly at 1000 metres, and on migration may attain 10000 metres or more. From their vantage point, they can see landmarks many kilometres away, and could detect smells and infrasound from more distant sources. It is possible that birds gather this information to form long-range mental maps, and use these to help them navigate on their vast migrations.

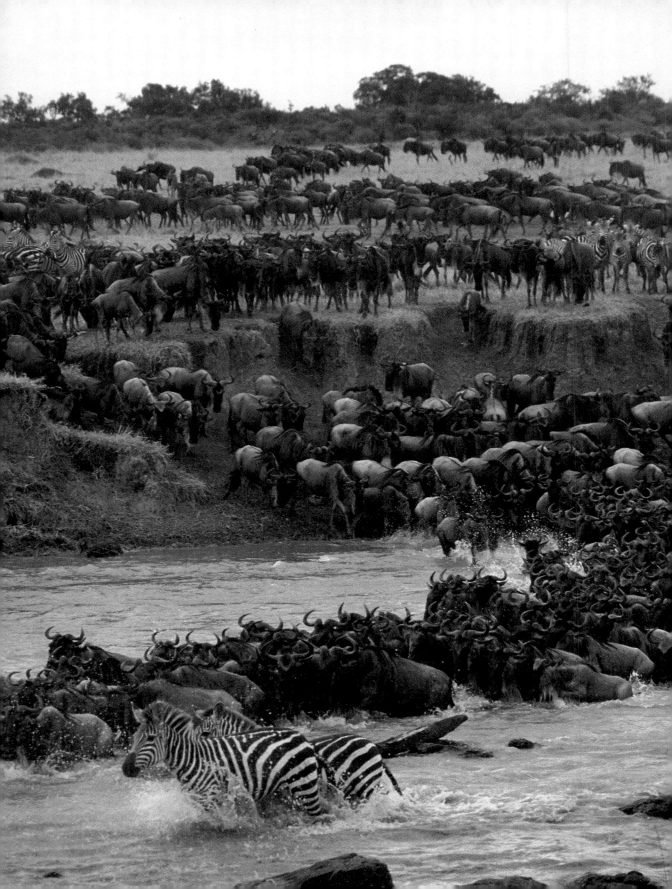

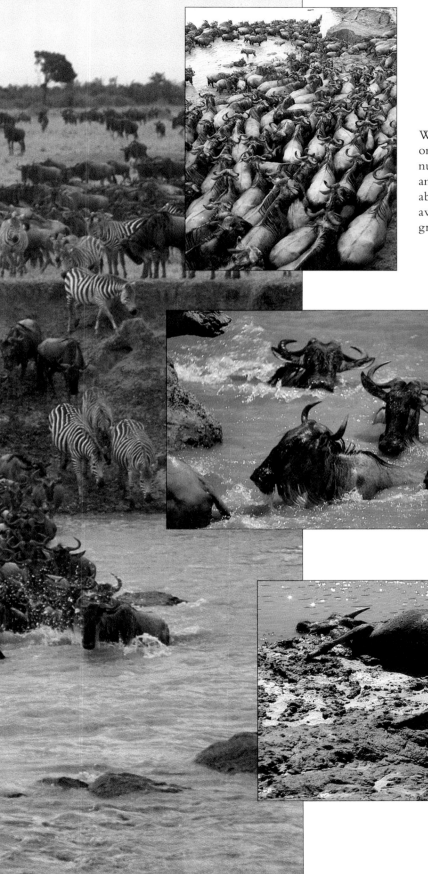

Wildebeest in the Serengeti embark on an annual migration in herds numbering tens of thousands of animals. The wildebeest may be able to sense the onset of rain far away, which stimulates fresh growth of grass in these areas.

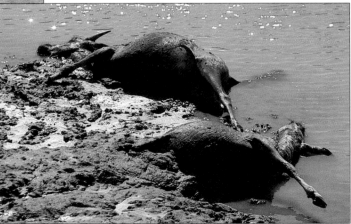

LONG-DISTANCE TRAVEL

Arctic terns spend the northern winter in the Antarctic, flying back to the far north in the spring to breed. They frequently return to the site where they were born, and use the same nest year after year. Their accuracy is almost certainly due to the mental maps they formed during their youthful explorations of their natal area.

Young swallows spend much of their time investigating their home range before they migrate to southern Africa for the winter. Earlier broods have more time to memorise the local area than later broods, and are more successful at finding their natal sites when they return in the following spring.

On their first migration, however, the young birds have to fly into the unknown. Some seem to use their parents or other birds as guides. Geese and swans travel in family groups along regular routes, while other birds fly in large flocks containing unrelated but experienced migrators. Similarly, the young travel alongside their parents in herds of migratory mammals, such as wildebeest and caribou. If a young animal is separated from its mother's herd, it becomes lost and wanders about aimlessly, unless it finds another herd to guide it.

Migrating herds and flocks seem to possess a collective wisdom which is handed down from the experienced to the young. However, migrating animals also have an innate tendency to move in a particular direction at certain times of the year. Experiments with white storks have shown how both instinct and learning play a part in navigating along migration routes. These large birds save energy during long-distance flights by using thermals to carry them up, and such rising columns of air only occur over the land. So, on their journey from Europe to Africa, the birds need to follow a route which avoids large expanses of sea. East European storks fly south-eastwards across the Bosphorus, while the west European population travels south-west across the Straits of Gibraltar. If east European storks are released in western Europe, they follow the local birds on their south-west journey. However, if their release is delayed until the local storks have departed, they follow their instinct and fly south-eastwards.

The cuckoo, reared by unrelated and often resident foster parents, has to find its own way to Africa. Birds such as this, which migrate alone, rely solely on instinct. Timing its departure by day length, the cuckoo sets off in a genetically predetermined direction, relying on its senses to maintain the correct compass bearing.

SENSORY BACK-UP SYSTEMS

We use mainly vision to find our way around, but we are not completely helpless in the dark because we can use touch and hearing to guide us. Similarly, migrating birds tend to rely on sight to navigate and have back-up systems for when this sense fails.

During the day, birds usually orient using their internal clock and the position of the sun. When the sun is hidden from our eyes by cloud, birds can detect any ultraviolet light that penetrates. Failing this, the pattern of polarised light in a small patch of blue sky will reveal the sun's location. At night the birds are guided by stars, such as the pole star, which indicates true north. Again, if this is hidden by cloud, the position of other stars can be used to pinpoint it. At some times, these visual cues are totally obscured, and then birds can fall back on their magnetic sense and even, possibly, smell and sound cues.

However, any sense can be rendered useless by circumstances or can give misleading information. Back-up systems lessen the risk of error, but cannot remove it entirely and even the birds' array of senses can be confused.

CONFUSED SENSES

The birds' preference for their visual rather than magnetic sense is probably due to the fact that the Earth's magnetic field often proves an unreliable guide. Magnetic anomalies can disorient migrating birds and seem to be responsible for the mass strandings of whales. Birds also have difficulty navigating during periods of high sunspot activity when magnetic storms sweep the Earth.

Visual cues may be more dependable than magnetic ones, but they are far from infallible. During their southward migrations of autumn, thousands of birds crash into lighthouses, apparently attracted by the artificial lights. It is possible that birds use the moon to navigate, and so orient southwards by flying towards the moon. On cloudy or moonless nights, a lighthouse beacon could be mistaken for the moon with disastrous results. Such a fate is common for moths which find their way around by flying at a fixed angle towards or away from the moon. This simple system worked well for millions of years until people created lights. Now, moths frequently try to maintain a constant angle towards artificial lights and so spiral inwards, often to their deaths.

Modern technology causes many other sensory disruptions. The enormous electric fields generated by power lines interfere with the sturgeon's delicate electrical navigation system. Sharks occasionally attack, and even sever, communication cables, probably because they mistake the cables' tiny electric fields for the body electricity of prey.

The ease with which even sophisticated sensory systems can be disturbed is exploited by many animals. The confusion created by human inventions is accidental, but in the natural world deliberate sensory deception is commonplace.

A TRICK OF THE LIGHT

Some animals use light to communicate with each other. For example, courting male fireflies emit bioluminescent signals and the females respond with a pattern of flashes.

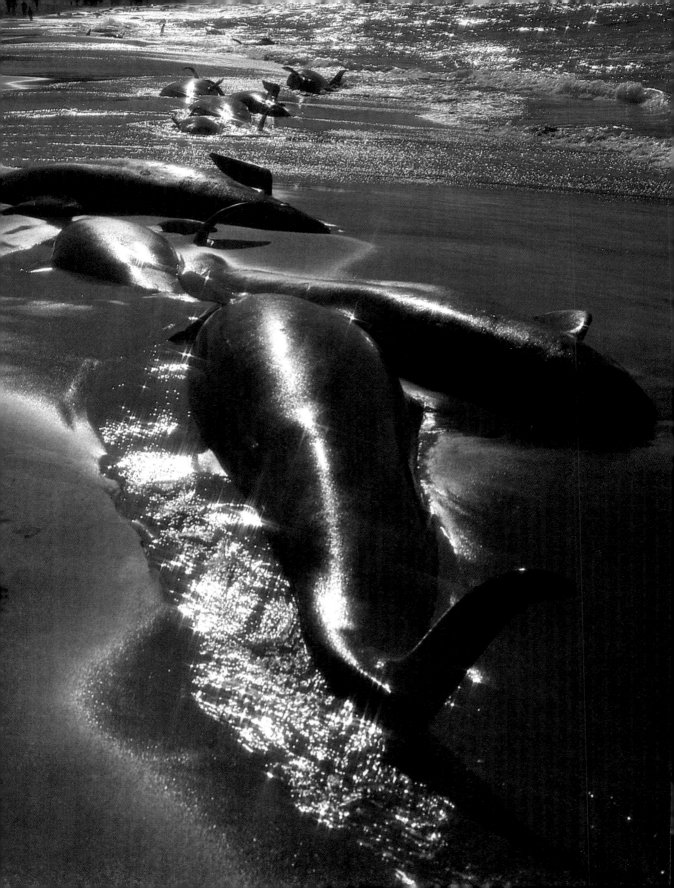

Strandings of whales (*opposite*) seem to occur when the animals follow magnetic contour lines which lead them to the shore.

Two examples of visual deception: The petal mantid (*below*) disguises itself as part of a flower to catch butterflies that are searching for nectar. As the Malayan stick insect (*right*) eats the leaf, its body covers the area it consumes. It is so similar to a leaf that it even has ribs and veins. In the picture the central rib is slightly mis-placed, making the match less than perfect.

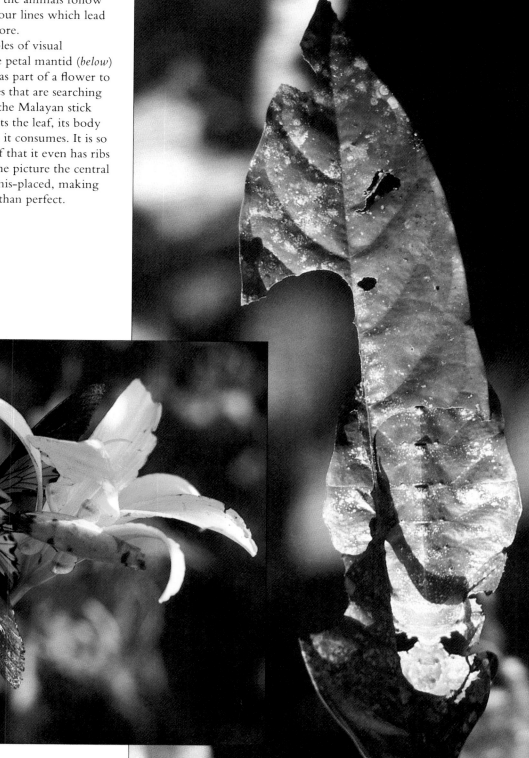

Each species has its own particular code of flashes to identify itself. A female carnivorous firefly, *Photuris*, turns this system to its advantage. By mimicking the flashcode used by the female of the related Photinus species, it attracts suitors which are then eaten by the femme fatale.

More commonly, animals rely on their eyes to find food, and both hunters and prey have evolved ways of confusing the visual sense of the other. The most impressive method is that employed by species of comb jelly, jellyfish, hydrozoans, arrow worms and other planktonic animals, which drift across the world's oceans. They are so transparent that they are virtually invisible to the human eye. Most higher animals cannot use this strategy because the pigment which screens the retina of the eye from strong light, and the contents of the stomach, reveal them. The Indian glass fish and many sea fish larvae attain a degree of invisibility, however, by concentrating their visible organs into a small area of the body. Another vanishing trick, favoured by human magicians and many fish, is to use mirrors. The fish's mirror-like scales reflect light and may cause the fish to 'disappear'.

An alternative disguise is to colour the body so that it blends in with the surroundings, as in the lichen-coloured wings of many moths, the green of leaf-eating caterpillars and the mottled brown plumage of ground-nesting birds. Many animals have adopted spots, stripes or other patterns to break up their body outlines and most are lighter underneath than on top to compensate for the shadow on the underside which would otherwise reveal them. Some are able to adapt to the changing hues brought by the seasons, such as the stoat and ptarmigan, which undergo a dramatic change to white in the winter. Others can vary their camouflage to match different surroundings, including the chameleon, and many frogs, fish and squid. Such transformations are achieved by the rapid movement of pigments within the cells or, in the case of the squid, the stretching of special pigment cells to form discs.

An equally effective strategy is to resemble another animal or plant, or an object. Some tropical butterflies imitate a leaf perfectly, even incorporating insect damage into their design. Many swallowtail caterpillars take on the appearance of bird droppings. When they grow too large for this disguise to be convincing, they moult and adopt a green camouflage instead.

Some bugs in Brazil achieve an uncanny resemblance to the head of an alligator, the only difference being their size, for the bugs are only a few centimetres long. The chrysalis of some African and Asian butterflies look exactly like the head of a rhesus monkey. Again, there is a difference in scale because the chrysalis is less than a centimetre long, but these diminutive mimics appear convincing to predatory birds. It seems that the eyes of hunting birds are much less conscious of depth than our own, and so a bird perceives the chrysalis as the face of a real monkey and flees.

An even more ingenious trick is practised by an orb-spider of the Andaman Islands. It collects together the remains of its insect prey and uses them to construct replicas of itself at various points on the web. This gives it safety in numbers if a bird attacks the web.

A remarkable number of visual deceptions have been discovered, probably because of the visual bias of human researchers. However, any sense can be fooled and tricks are now being unearthed in the rest of the sensory world.

DECEPTIVE SMELLS AND SOUNDS

Any animal which depends heavily on a particular sense lays itself open to deception. As was mentioned earlier, moths produce sexual scents to attract mates from several kilometres away. Spiders, such as the bolas spider, can imitate these scents and then ensnare the hapless suitors.

Ant and termite colonies rely on smell to identify intruders. Many insects, spiders and mites have managed to break through these chemical codes and slip unnoticed into colonies. For example, some staphylinid beetles release the characteristic odour of red ants and so live unmolested in the heart of the nest. They also emit another scent which stimulates the ants to feed them. Not content with this, they lay their eggs in the ants' brood chamber, and the beetle larvae thrive by consuming the young ants. The ants are so fooled by these deceptive scents that they will tend the beetle larvae in the midst of this destruction.

The most remarkable smell trickery, though, is practised by the *Harpagoxenus* ants of Scandinavia. These insects use slaves taken from the colonies of other species to maintain their nests. Suitable victims are found by a solitary scout which returns with a raiding party of several hundred ants. Instead of relying on brute force to enter the colony, they release a scent which sends the colony's guards into a fighting frenzy with each other. In the confusion, the raiding party captures workers and pupae using another scent.

The deathshead hawkmoth manages to sneak into a bee colony by using deceptive sounds. It mimics the thin piping squeak made by the queen bee and enters the nest to steal the honey.

A parasitic fly uses the pulsed sound created by male crickets to home in on a host and then lays its eggs in the cricket's body. Some males have learned to avoid this fate by sitting silently next to a singing cricket. They thus outwit the parasite and often successfully intercept a female.

Any deception will in time produce a counter-measure and may even initiate a sensory arms race. Such an escalation has occurred, for example, in the sound battle between bats and their prey.

THE SENSORY ARMS RACE

Many bats are almost completely reliant on their sophisticated echolocation system while hunting, and insects have evolved a host of ways of evading or clouding the bats' sound picture. Moths are covered with thick hairs, which absorb some of the bats' ultrasound. Lacewings, praying mantids and some moths can hear the bats' calls and swerve out of the way or close their wings and drop to the ground. Some distasteful moths emit an ultrasonic call, warning the bats that they are not worth catching. Other species produce blasts of ultrasound, apparently to confuse the bats' sonar. The blasts seem to be perceived by the bats as solid objects, causing the hunters to turn away.

These and other deceptive techniques have led some bats to develop a new system. The long-eared bat tunes its large parabolic ears to low frequencies and detects the wingbeats of its prey. However, many moths have found a way to counter this system as well. They have fine fringes at the tips of their wings to cut down the air turbulence responsible for flight noise.

Such adaptations take place throughout the natural world as animals develop ways of outwitting each other. They are responsible for the remarkable uses to which familiar senses are put, and for the evolution of supersenses.

INVESTIGATING SUPERSENSES

For many years, scientific explorations of the sensory worlds of other animals were limited by the bias of our own senses. Researchers tended to concentrate on our primary sense, vision, and in particular on the wavelengths of light which our eyes respond to. Much less attention was paid to hearing, and virtually none to sounds outside the narrow frequency range of our ears. Because of our under-utilised olfactory powers, the dominant role scents play in many animals' lives came as a revelation.

Over the last twenty years, however, investigations have revealed an amazing diversity of senses, and expanded dramatically our awareness of other animals' perceptions. As research continues, it is possible that our view of human powers may be extended too. For example, dowsers claim to be able to locate underground water and mineral deposits using a divining rod. Such deposits often occur in areas where faults, fractures or other features cause slight disturbances in the Earth's magnetic field. A magnetic sense is now known to be widespread in the animal kingdom, and it has been suggested that dowsers may be guided unconsciously by a sensitivity to magnetism.

Today, telepathy and other mysterious powers are called extra-sensory because they do not fit into our present framework of knowledge. However, the ability of some fish to produce force fields was incomprehensible until the discovery of electricity. In the future, more secrets may be unravelled showing that extra-sensory powers are no more mysterious, and no less remarkable than the supersenses so far discovered.

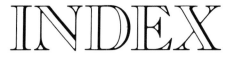

INDEX

Entries in bold type refer to an illustration.

PHOTOGRAPHIC ACKNOWLEDGEMENTS

AQUILA (Norman Fuller) page 90 top left; ARDEA pages 31 (P. Morris), 42 centre (P. Morris), 70 (Werner Curth), 94 and 135 (both François Gohier); BRUCE COLEMAN pages 2–3 (Norman Tomalin), 10 (Jeff Foott), 14 top (C. B. Frith), 18 bottom (Hans Reinhard), 19 (Jane Burton), 30–31 (Andy Purcell), 42 bottom (Jane Burton), 46 (Frieder Sauer), 47 bottom (Hans Reinhard), 66 (J. Cancalosi), 75 top (Kim Taylor), 91 (Frank Greenaway), 103 bottom (R. & M. Borland), 114 top (Frieder Sauer) & bottom (Jane Burton), 126–127 (A. J. Mobbs), 126 top (WWF/H. Jungius) and centre (N. G. Blake), 127 top & centre right (both Hans Reinhard), 127 centre left (J. Shaw), 131 top left (Roger Wilmshurst) & 134 (both Jeff Foott); DAILY TELEGRAPH (ESA Meteosat) page 27 bottom; NATURE PHOTOGRAPHERS page 99 bottom (Michael Gore); NHPA pages 42 top (Gérard Lacz) & 90 top right, bottom left & right (all Stephen Dalton); PLANET EARTH PICTURES pages 39 top (Ken Lucas) & centre bottom (Peter David), 47 top & centre (both John Lythgoe), 78–79 (James Hudnall), 78 bottom (Ocean Images/A. L. Giddings), 103 centre (Jonathan Scott), 130 bottom left (Cameron Read) & 154 (Tony Joyce); SURVIVAL ANGLIA pages 142–143 & 143 top (M. Kavanagh); UNIVERSITY OF BRISTOL, DEPT. OF VETERINARY SURGERY page 78 centre.

The remaining photographs were taken by John Downer.